FOODBORNE ILLNESS,
E. COLI AND SALMONELLA

PUBLIC HEALTH IN THE 21ST CENTURY

Additional books in this series can be found on Nova's website under the Series tab.

Additional E-books in this series can be found on Nova's website under the E-books tab.

FOODBORNE ILLNESS, E. COLI AND SALMONELLA

MARION LASKARIS

AND

FRED KOROL

EDITORS

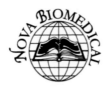

Nova Science Publishers, Inc.
New York

For permission to use material from this book please contact us:
Telephone 631-231-7269; Fax 631-231-8175
Web Site: http://www.novapublishers.com

NOTICE TO THE READER

The Publisher has taken reasonable care in the preparation of this book, but makes no expressed or implied warranty of any kind and assumes no responsibility for any errors or omissions. No liability is assumed for incidental or consequential damages in connection with or arising out of information contained in this book. The Publisher shall not be liable for any special, consequential, or exemplary damages resulting, in whole or in part, from the readers' use of, or reliance upon, this material. Any parts of this book based on government reports are so indicated and copyright is claimed for those parts to the extent applicable to compilations of such works.

Independent verification should be sought for any data, advice or recommendations contained in this book. In addition, no responsibility is assumed by the publisher for any injury and/or damage to persons or property arising from any methods, products, instructions, ideas or otherwise contained in this publication.

This publication is designed to provide accurate and authoritative information with regard to the subject matter covered herein. It is sold with the clear understanding that the Publisher is not engaged in rendering legal or any other professional services. If legal or any other expert assistance is required, the services of a competent person should be sought. FROM A DECLARATION OF PARTICIPANTS JOINTLY ADOPTED BY A COMMITTEE OF THE AMERICAN BAR ASSOCIATION AND A COMMITTEE OF PUBLISHERS.

Additional color graphics may be available in the e-book version of this book.

Library of Congress Cataloging-in-Publication Data

The Library of Congress has cataloged the original edition of this title under LCCN 2010015624 and 2008008040

ISBN 978-1-62100-052-5

Published by Nova Science Publishers, Inc. † New York

Contents

Preface

Health officials monitor and investigate foodborne illness in a number of ways. Surveillance is used to track trends in the incidence of several common bacterial and parasitic foodborne illnesses. Tracking of outbreaks of foodborne illness helps improve approaches to investigation. Genetic "fingerprinting" is also used to identify infections from a common source, including large multistate outbreaks. Collectively, these tools shed light on the burden of foodborne illness in the U.S., and ways to decrease it. This book examines several systems to monitor foodborne illnesses, discussing their strengths and the gaps that remain in understanding the burden of foodborne illness in the United States, with a focus on E. coli and salmonella.

Chapter 1- The 111th Congress is considering legislation to revise the U.S. food safety system, focusing primarily on those laws and programs administered by the Food and Drug Administration (FDA) within the Department of Health and Human Services (HHS). The House has passed a comprehensive bill, H.R. 2749, and the Senate Committee on Health, Education, Labor, and Pensions has reported its comprehensive proposal, S. 510. The ultimate goal of both bills is to reduce the burden of foodborne illness, which is a considerable and persistent public health problem in the United States. However, an understanding of the true burden of illness caused by foodborne hazards, the risks associated with various types of foods, and the types of regulatory and other approaches that can effectively address these problems has been elusive.

Chapter 2- In September 2006, government officials were alerted to an outbreak of E. coliO157:H7 infections associated with the consumption of tainted fresh spinach. For several weeks, the Food and Drug Administration (FDA) and the Centers for Disease Control and Prevention (CDC) investigated the situation as additional cases were identified nearly daily. This report details the events as they unfolded, and includes the number of cases, the detection of the first case, and the process by which relevant agencies acted as subsequent cases were reported. This report will be updated in response to any further developments.

Chapter 3- *Escherichia coli* (abbreviated as *E. coli*) are a large and diverse group of bacteria. Although most strains of *E. coli* are harmless, others can make you sick. Some kinds of *E. coli* can cause diarrhea, while others cause urinary tract infections, respiratory illness and pneumonia, and other illnesses. Still other kinds of *E. coli* are used as markers for water contamination—so you might hear about *E. coli* being found in drinking water, which are not themselves harmful, but indicate the water is contaminated. It does get a bit confusing—even to microbiologists.

Chapter 4- Shiga toxin–producing *Escherichia coli* (STEC) are a leading cause of bacterial enteric infections in the United States. Prompt, accurate diagnosis of STEC infection is important because appropriate treatment early in the course of infection might decrease the risk for serious complications such as renal damage and improve overall patient outcome. In addition, prompt laboratory identification of STEC strains is essential for detecting new and emerging serotypes, for effective and timely outbreak responses and control measures, and for monitoring trends in disease epidemiology. Guidelines for laboratory identification of STEC infections by clinical laboratories were published in 2006 (1). This report provides comprehensive and detailed recommendations for STEC testing by clinical laboratories, including the recommendation that all stools submitted for routine testing from patients with acute community-acquired diarrhea (regardless of patient age, season of the year, or presence or absence of blood in the stool) be simultaneously cultured for *E. coli* O157:H7 (O157 STEC) and tested with an assay that detects Shiga toxins to detect non- O157 STEC. The report also includes detailed procedures for specimen selection, handling, and transport; a review of culture and nonculture tests for STEC detection; and clinical considerations and recommendations for management of patients with STEC infection. Improving the diagnostic accuracy of STEC infection by clinical laboratories should ensure prompt diagnosis and treatment of these infections in patients and increase detection of STEC outbreaks in the community.

Chapter 5- Between January and April 2009, a foodborne illness outbreak linked to *Salmonella* resulted in one of the largest food safety recalls ever in the United States. The source of the outbreak was linked to one peanut processor handling less than 2 percent of the U.S. peanut supply, but the scope of the recalls was magnified because the processed peanut products were used as ingredients in more than 3,900 products. Although consumer purchases of peanut-containing products initially slowed as the scope of the recalls spread, retail purchases returned to normal within several months and the total volume of peanuts processed during the 2008/09 (August-July) marketing year increased slightly from that of the previous year. These developments suggest that the recalls will not have a lasting impact on peanut demand and production.

In: Foodborne Illness, E. coli and Salmonella   ISBN: 978-1-62100-052-5
Editors: M. Laskaris and F. Korol   © 2011 Nova Science Publishers, Inc.

Chapter 1

Food Safety: Foodborne Illness and Selected Recalls of FDA-Regulated Foods

Sarah A. Lister and Geoffrey S. Becker

Summary

The 111th Congress is considering legislation to revise the U.S. food safety system, focusing primarily on those laws and programs administered by the Food and Drug Administration (FDA) within the Department of Health and Human Services (HHS). The House has passed a comprehensive bill, H.R. 2749, and the Senate Committee on Health, Education, Labor, and Pensions has reported its comprehensive proposal, S. 510. The ultimate goal of both bills is to reduce the burden of foodborne illness, which is a considerable and persistent public health problem in the United States. However, an understanding of the true burden of illness caused by foodborne hazards, the risks associated with various types of foods, and the types of regulatory and other approaches that can effectively address these problems has been elusive.

Public health officials monitor and investigate foodborne illnesses in a number of ways. For example, active surveillance is used to track trends in the incidence of several common bacterial and parasitic foodborne illnesses. Outbreaks of foodborne illness are tracked to help improve approaches to investigation and to identify the foods that cause illnesses, among other things. Genetic "fingerprinting" is used to identify infections from a common source, including large multistate outbreaks, and can also help identify the foods that cause illnesses. These systems are administered jointly by various federal agencies, in partnership with state health officials. Collectively, these tools and others can shed light on the burden of foodborne illness in the United States, and ways to decrease it. However, these systems also have two significant shortcomings. First, because they monitor a limited number of known food safety threats, and because foodborne illnesses are substantially underreported, these systems do not, individually or collectively, capture the magnitude of foodborne illness that occurs each year. Second, these systems often detect or track the contaminant that causes illness, rather than the type of food that was contaminated, although it is the latter that government officials actually regulate.

Consumers and the media often focus on recalls—particularly those that are extensive and/or that involve widely consumed products—as indicators of the safety of the U.S. food supply. In many but certainly not all cases, products subject to a recall may have sickened or killed people or other animals. It is not always clear, however, how useful recall data are as a measure of the burden of foodborne illness or the effectiveness of federal food safety programs. For example, does a relatively high number of recalls signify a failure of the system to keep unsafe products from being consumed? Or is it actually an indication that the safety net is working by finding and getting tainted products off the market? Conversely, is a relatively low number of recalls an indication of the system's effectiveness, or simply of not reporting or finding all defective food products? Because of these questions, caution should be exercised in using recall data as the basis for concluding that certain changes are needed in the nation's food safety systems.

This report describes several systems to monitor foodborne illnesses, discussing their strengths and the gaps that remain in understanding the burden of foodborne illness in the United States. Next, this report presents recent data on more serious recalls of FDA-regulated foods, also discussing the strengths and gaps associated with the information. Finally, this report describes three recent foodborne outbreaks that led to nationwide recalls of FDA-regulated foods: (1) *Salmonella* in peanut products, (2) melamine in pet foods and dairy products, and (3) *E. coli* in spinach. Following each description are discussions of associated policy issues, and, if applicable, how these issues are addressed in food safety legislation pending before the 111th Congress. Descriptions of selected authorities in the Federal Food, Drug, and Cosmetic Act (FFDCA), FDA's principal food safety law, are provided in the Appendix.

Introduction

The Government Accountability Office (GAO) has identified as many as 15 federal agencies that collectively administer at least 30 laws related to food safety.[1] The Food and Drug Administration (FDA) within the Department of Health and Human Services (HHS) and the Food Safety and Inspection Service (FSIS) within the U.S. Department of Agriculture (USDA) together comprise the majority of both the total funding and the total staffing of the federal government's food regulatory system. FDA has lead responsibility for ensuring the safety of all human and animal foods except those from the major meat and poultry species, catfish, and some egg products. These latter types of foods are within the purview of FSIS. According to GAO, FDA-regulated foods account for 80% of at-home U.S. food spending.[2] In addition to federal activities, states may play a substantial role in food facility inspections, outbreak investigations, and other food safety activities, particularly with respect to FDA-regulated foods.

The 111th Congress is considering legislation to revise the U.S. food safety system, focusing primarily on those laws and programs administered by FDA. Both the House and Senate have introduced comprehensive bills that address a number of perceived problems with the current food safety system. The House passed H.R. 2749, the Food Safety Enhancement Act of 2009, on July 30, 2009. The Senate Committee on Health, Education, Labor, and Pensions has reported S. 510, the FDA Food Safety Modernization Act. The bills cover much of the same material, although they differ somewhat in their specific approaches. Among other things, both bills would expand registration requirements for food facilities and require facilities to implement food safety plans based on assessments of risk. Also, both bills would require FDA to conduct periodic safety inspections, expand the agency's access to industry records, and allow the agency to mandate that companies conduct recalls of unsafe products. Both bills would also set new standards for produce safety and place more scrutiny on imported foods.

The FDA faces considerable challenges in assuring the safety of the foods for which it is responsible. The complexity of the food distribution system is steadily increasing. Processed foods, in particular, may contain dozens of ingredients with domestic and imported origins. Similarly, a contaminated ingredient may find its way into dozens of seemingly unrelated products, including foods for both humans and animals. The ultimate goal of the House and Senate food safety bills is to reduce foodborne illness, which is a considerable and persistent public health problem in the United States.

However, a comprehensive understanding of the burden of illness caused by foodborne hazards, the risks posed by different types of foods, and the types of safeguards that can effectively address these problems has been elusive.

This report describes several systems to monitor foodborne illnesses and define the burden of this public health problem in the United States. Next, this report presents recent data on more serious recalls of FDA-regulated foods. Finally, this report describes three recent foodborne outbreaks that led to nationwide recalls of FDA-regulated foods: (1) *Salmonella* in peanut products, (2) melamine in pet foods and dairy products, and (3) *E. coli* in spinach. Following each description are discussions of associated policy issues, and, if applicable, how these issues are addressed in the food safety legislation pending before the 111th Congress. Descriptions of selected authorities in the Federal Food, Drug, and Cosmetic Act (FFDCA), FDA's principal food safety law, are provided in the Appendix. Like the bills under consideration, the main focus of this report is on the FDA and its authorities and approaches to assure food safety.

The Burden of Foodborne Illness

Overview and Estimates

Health officials monitor and investigate foodborne illness in a number of ways. For example, surveillance is used to track trends in the incidence of several common bacterial and parasitic foodborne illnesses. Tracking of outbreaks of foodborne illness helps improve approaches to investigation, among other things. Genetic "fingerprinting" is used to identify infections from a common source, including large multistate outbreaks.

Collectively, these tools shed light on the burden of foodborne illness in the United States, and ways to decrease it. However, these tools also have two significant shortcomings. First, because they monitor a limited number of known food safety threats, and because foodborne illnesses are substantially underreported, these systems do not, individually or collectively, capture the magnitude of foodborne illness that occurs each year. Second, they often detect the contaminant that causes illness, rather than the type of food that was contaminated, although it is the latter that government officials actually regulate. These concepts are discussed below, followed by descriptions of three key federal foodborne illness monitoring systems: FoodNet active surveillance of individual cases of foodborne illness; surveillance of foodborne disease outbreaks; and PulseNet genetic "fingerprinting" of certain foodborne pathogens. Key definitions are provided in a text box, below.

Because the existing foodborne illness surveillance systems do not identify all cases of foodborne illness, health officials can only estimate the true burden of illness in the population. In 1999, the Centers for Disease Control and Prevention (CDC) published such an estimate for the United States, saying that on average, about 76 million people become sick, 325,000 are hospitalized, and 5,000 die each year from foodborne illnesses caused by one or more of a number of microbial pathogens and other contaminants.[3] The authors noted that most foodborne illnesses are not reported to authorities, and are therefore not reflected in foodborne illness surveillance data.[4] They also reported that

> many pathogens transmitted through food are also spread through water or from person to person, thus obscuring the role of foodborne transmission. Finally, some proportion of foodborne illness is caused by pathogens or agents that have not yet been identified and thus cannot be diagnosed. The importance of this final factor cannot be overstated. Many of the pathogens of greatest concern today (e.g., *Campylobacter jejuni*, [E. coli] O157:H7, *Listeria monocytogenes*, [and] *Cyclospora cayetanensis*) were not recognized as causes of foodborne illness just 20 years ago.[5]

CDC's estimate was derived from a variety of data sources, dating from 1997 and earlier. The agency is in the process of revising the estimate.

Definitions: Foodborne Illness Investigation

Active Surveillance: Active surveillance means that CDC and state health officials follow up with physicians, laboratories, and others to assure completeness of reporting. Active surveillance is labor- and time-intensive.

Attribution: Determining, through investigation, the type of food vehicle responsible for transmitting etiologic agents that cause foodborne illness.

Cause: Referring to the cause of a foodborne illness or outbreak may be confusing, as it could refer either to the etiology or to the vehicle. Also, a food production or handling practice could be implicated in an outbreak investigation, and could also be referred to as a "cause."

Etiology: The pathogen (bacteria, viruses, parasites or fungi), toxin, or other contaminant that causes illnesses in humans or other animals. These contaminants may be referred to as *etiologic agents*.

Genetic "fingerprinting": Refers to several approaches to describe the specific make-up of a bacterial pathogen, such as its genetic material, cell wall components, or other features, in order to distinguish related strains from other strains. For example, the PulseNet system uses pulsed-field gel electrophoresis (PFGE) to break apart and separate bands of bacterial DNA. Identical banding patterns usually mean that the strains are genetically related, and that they arose from common origins and/or were transmitted through a common vehicle. This approach allows health officials to, for example, quickly distinguish among many thousands of strains of *Salmonella* that cause illness each year, to see if one of them is responsible for illnesses identified across jurisdictions.

Outbreak: A foodborne disease outbreak is not defined in law or in regulation. In public health practice, a foodborne disease outbreak is defined as "the occurrence of two or more cases of a similar illness resulting from the ingestion of a common food." As a practical matter, particularly for less serious hazards, outbreak investigations are rarely launched when only two people are affected, although there are exceptions, such as for botulism.

Passive Surveillance: Unlike active surveillance, passive surveillance does not involve efforts to validate the completeness of reporting. As a result, under-reporting is usually more of a concern than with active surveillance.

Vehicle: The type of food that carries or transmits an etiologic agent.

Source: Adapted by CRS from CDC, "Surveillance for Foodborne-Disease Outbreaks: United States, 1998–2002," *MMWR*, vol. 55 (Surveillance Summary 10), pp. 1-34, November 10, 2006; and CDC, "Overview of CDC Food Safety Activities and Programs," http://www.cdc.gov/foodsafety/fsactivities.htm.

As noted earlier, foodborne illness surveillance generally identifies illnesses by their *etiology*, that is, the pathogen or other contaminant responsible for illness, such as *Salmonella* or the toxin that causes botulism. It is more difficult to identify the *vehicle*, that is, the type of food that bears the contaminant. For example, foodborne illness surveillance systems track cases of human *Salmonella* infection. It can be difficult to attribute these infections to one or more of a variety of possible vehicles, which may include poultry, eggs, produce, and dairy products, among others. When a vehicle is identified, it can then be difficult to identify the practice that caused the contamination, such as an on-farm or processing practice, or cross-contamination in the home or food-service establishment. Because regulators are responsible for the safety of food vehicles and food production and handling practices, and not the etiologies *per se*, the gap between identification of an illness or outbreak and implication of a food vehicle and/or practice remains a substantial challenge in reducing the burden of foodborne illness in the United States.

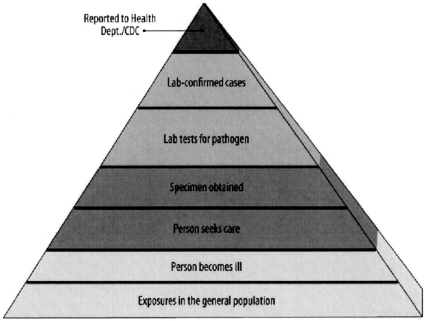

Source: Adapted by CRS from CDC, "FoodNet Surveillance–Burden of Illness Pyramid," http://www.cdc.gov/FoodNet/surveillance_pages/burden_pyramid.htm.

Figure 1. Pyramid Showing Burden of Foodborne Illness.

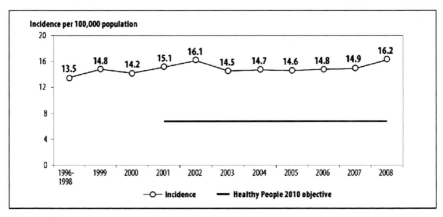

Source: Prepared by CRS from FoodNet annual reports, http://www.cdc.gov/mmwr/; and Healthy People 2010, Ch. 10, Food Safety, http://www.healthypeople.gov /Document/HTML/Volume1/10Food.htm.

Notes: According to CDC, the increased incidence (cases per 100,000 population) for *Salmonella* in 2008 was not statistically significant when compared with the rates for the previous three years. The 1996-1998 *Salmonella* incidence is a three-year average, as published by CDC. The Healthy People 2010 objective for *Salmonella* is to halve the incidence from the 1997 baseline of 13.7 cases per 100,000 to 6.8 cases per 100,000 by 2010.

Figure 2. Incidence of Human *Salmonella* Infections in the United States, 1996–2008 From FoodNet Active Surveillance of Laboratory-Confirmed Cases.

Following are presentations of three important monitoring systems for foodborne illness: FoodNet active surveillance of certain pathogens; passive surveillance of foodborne disease outbreaks; and PulseNet genetic "fingerprinting" of certain foodborne bacteria.[6] These and other monitoring systems together provide information about the nature of foodborne illnesses in the United States, and, increasingly, information about the means to prevent them.

FoodNet: Active Surveillance of Foodborne Illness

Since 1996, the *FoodNet* system has been used to monitor the incidence of certain foodborne illnesses. FoodNet is a population-based active surveillance system chiefly administered by CDC in partnership with FDA, USDA, and 10 states.[7] FoodNet tracks the incidence of individual laboratory-confirmed infections caused by several bacteria and parasites, in sites in the 10 states. Because FoodNet tracks only laboratory-confirmed infections, it does not capture foodborne illnesses that do not involve a health care visit, testing with a positive result, and reporting of that result. Figure 1 presents the "burden of illness" pyramid, showing that FoodNet data capture only the "tip of the iceberg." Also, the bacteria and parasites monitored by the FoodNet system account for only a portion of the causes of foodborne illness each year.

For the reasons noted above, FoodNet does not provide information about the overall burden of foodborne illness in the United States. Also, FoodNet data do not capture information (if it is known) about the food vehicle(s) that caused reported illnesses.[8] However, because FoodNet monitors illnesses in the same population and in the same way from year to year, capturing most or all laboratory-confirmed cases through active surveillance, the system can be used to track trends in the incidence of foodborne illness. FoodNet data can indicate whether the problem of illnesses caused by a specific pathogen appears to be getting better or worse over time, which can provide general information about the effectiveness of food safety programs, among other things. Prior to the implementation of FoodNet, it was not possible to track the monitored foodborne illnesses in this way.

Based on FoodNet data, CDC reported that in 2008 the incidence of several of the illnesses under surveillance since 1996 had reached a plateau, instead of declining, and that national Healthy People 2010 (HP2010) health targets for these illnesses may not be met.[9] For example, Figure 2 presents the FoodNet incidence of *Salmonella* infections from 1996 through 2008, and the HP2010 target. CDC has said that of all the FoodNet pathogens, the incidence of *Salmonella* is farthest from the HP2010 target, and that meeting the target in the future will likely require new approaches to prevention.[10] CDC also commented on efforts at FSIS to reduce levels of *Salmonella* contamination in poultry, a common vehicle for *Salmonella* infection. But CDC also noted the growing recognition that several types of food vehicles regulated by FDA, such as peanut products and leafy greens, may also contribute considerably to the burden of illnesses caused by the FoodNet pathogens, including *Salmonella*.

Passive Surveillance of Foodborne Disease Outbreaks

In addition to FoodNet, CDC also partners with FDA, USDA, and state and local health officials to coordinate national passive surveillance of foodborne disease outbreaks (FBDOs), which are groups of illnesses that result from a common exposure.[11] Outbreaks may involve as few as two or as many as thousands of people. Outbreak reporting differs from FoodNet reporting in several ways. First, FoodNet tracks individual cases of illness only for a handful of specific etiologies, such as *Salmonella*, and only when infections are laboratory-confirmed. In contrast, for some outbreaks the etiology is never identified; the recognition of an outbreak may hinge only on the finding of common symptoms among individuals with an obvious common exposure. For example, if a group of people experience acute vomiting after eating at the same function, and no etiology is identified, states authorities could report the incident to CDC as an outbreak, but FoodNet would not capture any of the cases.[12] Also, most foodborne illnesses are "sporadic;" that is, they are not associated with outbreaks. Finally, as with individual cases of illness, many outbreaks, particularly those that are small, are not reported to authorities. Therefore, outbreak data provide limited information about the incidence or overall burden of foodborne illness.

A strength of outbreak data is that it may provide attribution information that is not captured by FoodNet. Investigating outbreaks may allow health officials to attribute them to specific types of foods and/or food handling practices, as well as to identify the types of techniques that are most effective in responding to and controlling a FBDO. A food safety advocacy group maintains a database of foodborne outbreaks (involving two or more people) in the United States for which the outbreak was attributed to a specific food vehicle(s), compiled largely from CDC and state health department outbreak listings, reports by the CDC's Foodborne Outbreak Response and Surveillance Unit, and peer-reviewed journal articles.[13] The group identified a total of 5,778 outbreaks of illness linked to specific foods between 1990 and 2006, reporting hundreds of outbreaks each attributed to seafood, meat, poultry, produce, and eggs. It also noted the problem associated with attribution of outbreaks to multi-ingredient foods, namely, that it can be more difficult to identify the contaminated ingredient in these situations.

In summary, FBDO data capture passive reports of outbreaks based on symptoms of foodborne illness among groups of people. Reported outbreaks may or may not be accompanied by information about an identified etiology and/or an attributed food or food handling practice. Outbreaks vary considerably in size, from small ones linked to social gatherings, to large ones involving commercial products consumed by thousands of people across the country. FBDO data may be most useful when considered qualitatively (e.g., saying that produce continues to be a source of multiple large FBDOs each year), but may not support quantitative conclusions (e.g., saying that produce is a leading cause of foodborne illness, compared with other vehicles).[14]

PulseNet: Genetic "Fingerprinting"

In the last two decades, technologies to link foodborne illnesses that have a common bacterial etiology have revolutionized the ability to identify large multistate outbreaks and mount an urgent response.[15] The PulseNet program, coordinated by CDC, links state and local health departments and federal agencies (including CDC, FDA, and FSIS) to a common database to determine whether bacteria that are associated with illnesses or found on foods are related. By its nature, PulseNet analyzes only laboratory-confirmed illnesses caused by several specific pathogens.

Although the PulseNet system can greatly improve the speed of detection of an outbreak, the tools used subsequently to attribute the responsible food vehicle(s) remain cumbersome. Epidemiologists often must still rely on time-consuming patient interviews. Especially for those foodborne infections with long incubation periods, patients' recollection of foods eaten may be imperfect. Also, if interviews suggest a suspicious subset of foods, the foods may no longer be available for testing. In addition, especially for FDA-regulated foods, information about common contaminants that may be present during production and in commerce, as well as how to test for them, is limited.[16] For these reasons, attribution of illnesses and outbreaks to a specific food vehicle remains a significant challenge.

FDA-Announced Food Recalls

With the exception of infant formula, FDA does not have the authority to order a recall of an unsafe or potentially unsafe food.[17] Rather, the agency relies on food companies to voluntarily recall adulterated, misbranded, or otherwise unsafe products, either on their own initiative or upon regulators' request. Some in the food industry assert that the industry rarely if ever fails to conduct a recall when necessary, although the U.S. Government Accountability Office (GAO) has identified some instances of non-cooperation.[18]

FDA has stated that a company recall is generally the most effective current means for protecting consumers, but the FDA's principal statute, the Federal Food, Drug, and Cosmetic Act (FFDCA), does provide the agency with other legal enforcement tools, such as the power to seize adulterated and misbranded products. Such tools can be employed if a recall is not undertaken or is found to be ineffective.

A recall is "a firm's removal or correction of a marketed product that the [FDA] considers to be in violation of the laws it administers and against which the agency would initiate legal action, e.g., seizure."[19] The FDA categorizes recalls into three classes, as follows:

- Class I recalls, the most serious, involve "situation[s] in which there is a reasonable probability that the use of, or exposure to, a violative product will cause serious adverse health consequences or death."
- Class II recalls involve "situation[s] in which use of, or exposure to, a violative product may cause temporary or medically reversible adverse health consequences or where the probability of serious adverse health consequences is remote."
- Class III recalls involve "situation[s] in which use of, or exposure to, a violative product is not likely to cause adverse health consequences."[20]

FDA compiles information about recalls primarily via two publicly accessible formats. The first is a regularly updated listing, in reverse chronological order, of each major recall or related action regarding products it regulates (i.e., drugs, biologics, medical devices, cosmetics, and most foods).[21] This listing consists primarily of Class I recalls. Each item on the list is hot-linked to a press release announcing the recall, with additional details on the type of product, the reason for the recall, its geographical extent, and other basic information. The agency currently offers an online archive for these recalls dating back to 2004, and the database is searchable. Second, FDA publishes weekly enforcement reports that generally contain the same information, also dating back to 2004.[22] The information in these reports appears to be less current than that in the first source, but is said by FDA to be more complete in that it includes all Class I, II, and III recalls.

Recalls—particularly those involving large numbers of widely consumed products—cause consumers to question not only the safety records of the recalling companies but also the ability of health officials to protect the food supply. In many, but certainly not all, cases, products subject to a recall may have sickened or killed people or animals. It is not clear, however, how useful FDA recall data are as a measure of the burden of foodborne illness or the effectiveness of federal food safety programs. For example, does a relatively high number of recalls signify a failure of the system to keep unsafe products from being consumed, or does it indicate that the safety system is working by finding unsafe products and removing them from the market? Conversely, is a relatively low number of recalls an indication of the system's effectiveness, or simply of not finding and/or reporting all unsafe food products? Because of these questions, care should be exercised in using recall data as the basis for evaluating the effectiveness of food safety efforts. With these caveats in mind, CRS presents, in Table 1, the total number of Class I and Class II recalls of FDA-regulated foods for each of FY2005 through FY2009, by type of product, as categorized by FDA. (The data do not include Class III recalls, which, according to the definition, are not likely to involve problems that could cause foodborne illness.)

These tabulations do not include the several hundred recalls, which occurred during the same time period, of various meat and poultry products regulated by FSIS. Like FDA, FSIS also does not have mandatory recall authority and thus relies on private firms to voluntarily withdraw products from commerce when problems arise. However, FSIS's recall policies and its other enforcement authorities differ from those of FDA in some other ways.[23]

The data in Table 1 show a spike in the number of products recalled in the first 11 months of FY2009. Most of this increase appears to be linked to two major food safety incidents in 2009. The first was a widespread outbreak of *Salmonella* linked to consumption of contaminated peanut ingredients from a single company's plants. Peanut butter, peanut paste, and related ingredients from this company, Peanut Corporation of America (PCA), were used by hundreds of other companies in thousands of products that collectively constituted hundreds of the FY2009 recalls. In Table 1, increases in the following categories are likely to reflect PCA-related products that were recalled: bakery products, doughs, bakery mixes, icings; nuts and edible seeds; snack food items; chocolate and cocoa products; ice cream and related products; and candy without chocolate. See the subsequent section of this report, "*Salmonella* Outbreak from Peanut Products (2008–2009)," for more information about this recall.

The second incident—*Salmonella* contamination of pistachio nuts that were also provided to many other companies by a single supplier—led to another 100 or more recalls. Although the number of peanut- and pistachio-related recalls appears to be particularly high, multiple recalls traced to a single common problem source are not surprising given the organization of the U.S. food system, where a single supplier may provide products or ingredients to hundreds of processors and distributors nationwide.

**Table 1. Recalls of FDA-Regulated Foods, by Product
Type, FY2005-FY2009**

Product Type	FY2005	FY2006	FY2007	FY2008	FY2009	Totals	% of all Recalls FY2005-FY2009
Bakery products, doughs, bakery mixes, icings	73	42	62	85	164	426	13.4%
Multiple food dinners, gravies, sauces, specialties	137	16	38	44	92	327	10.3%
Fishery/seafood products	76	56	41	59	37	269	8.5%
Nuts and edible seeds	15	5	24	9	216	269	8.5%
Fruit and fruit products	36	25	81	72	23	237	7.5%
Snack food items (flour, meal, vegetable base)	10	7	16	7	183	223	7.0%
Chocolate and cocoa products	10	19	29	32	127	217	6.8%
Vitamins, minerals, proteins, unconventional diet	41	12	52	32	69	206	6.5%
Vegetables and vegetable products	39	35	25	33	50	182	5.7%
Spices, flavors, salts	33	3	3	11	61	111	3.5%
Ice cream and related products	12	6	5	15	60	98	3.1%
Candy without chocolate, candy specialties, gum	11	7	4	5	69	96	3.0%
Prepared salad products	0	21	8	40	3	72	2.3%
Dietary conventional foods and meal replacements	7	7	2	3	42	61	1.9%
Milk, butter, dried milk products	1	4	3	3	46	57	1.8%
Cheese and cheese products	5	9	7	11	15	47	1.5%

Product Type	FY2005	FY2006	FY2007	FY2008	FY2009	Totals	% of all Recalls FY2005-FY2009
Soft drinks and waters	4	2	13	10	3	32	1.0%
Cereal preparations, breakfast foods	1	1	3	10	13	28	0.9%
Coffee and tea	5	10	3	1	7	26	0.8%
Soups	4	5	2	7	8	26	0.8%
Dressings and condiments	6	4	4	6	4	24	0.8%
Gelatin, rennet, pudding mixes, pie fillings	1	4	13	0	5	23	0.7%
Baby (infant and junior) food products	3	5	7	4	0	19	0.6%
Macaroni and noodle products	12	3	1	0	1	17	0.5%
Vegetable protein products (simulated meats)	10	2	0	5	0	17	0.5%
Whole grains, milled grain products, starch	2	8	5	1	0	16	0.5%
Filled/imitation milk products	1	0	6	1	4	12	0.4%
Meat, meat products, and poultry	0	2	0	1	6	9	0.3%
Beverage bases	0	0	0	0	8	8	0.3%
Food sweeteners (nutritive)	1	0	6	0	0	7	0.2%
Eggs and egg products	1	2	0	1	2	6	0.2%
Other	0	1	0	2	1	4	0.1%
TOTAL FOOD RECALLS	**557**	**323**	**463**	**510**	**1319**	**3172**	**100.0%**

Source: Prepared by CRS based on data provided by FDA via e-mail, August 31, 2009.

Notes: FY2009 is for 11 months (through August). Figures are counts of recall announcements, which can involve more than one recalled product. Includes Class I and Class II recalls. Does not include several hundred recalls that occurred during the same time period involving meat and poultry products regulated by FSIS.

Also of note in Table 1 is that nine food product types, out of nearly 35 categories logged by the FDA, accounted for approximately 75% of all recalls during the FY2005-2009 period.[24] The leading category (as designated by FDA) was bakery products, doughs, bakery mixes, and icings, which accounted for 13.4% of all recalls. This was followed by the category of multiple food dinners, gravies, sauces, specialties, with 10.3% of all recalls during FY2005-2009. Snack foods and chocolate products, respectively, constituted 7% and 6.8% of all recalls. It may not be surprising that all four of these categories involve diverse product lines that combine many different ingredients. The other five categories among the nine leaders were fishery and seafood products, and nuts and edible seeds, each with 8.5% of the total recalls; fruit and fruit products, 7.5%; vitamins, minerals, proteins, and unconventional dietary items, 6.5%; and vegetables and vegetable products, 5.7%.

Selected FDA Food Recalls: Information and Implications

Following are discussions of three recalls involving FDA-regulated foods. These recalls were selected by CRS for their scope, the interest they generated among the press and the public, and their illustration of several policy issues under debate in pending food safety legislation (H.R. 2749 and S. 510). Following a description of each recall are discussions of selected issues and brief mentions of the relationship to pending legislation, when applicable. Descriptions of selected current authorities in the FFDCA are provided in the **Appendix**. This CRS report does not provide comprehensive information about the House and Senate food safety bills or the differences between their approaches to the policy issues discussed here.

Salmonella Outbreak from Peanut Products (2008–2009)[25]

Overview

One of the largest food recalls in U.S. history began on January 11, 2009, when King Nut Companies announced it was recalling peanut butter it distributed to food service institutions. The company said *Salmonella* had been found in a five-pound tub of the product, manufactured for the firm by Peanut

Corporation of America (PCA). The first PCA recall of its own products was announced on January 13, 2009, and by the end of the month had been extended several times to include all PCA peanuts and peanut products (including meal, butter, paste, and granulated). Over the ensuing months, the number of PCA-related recalls grew to approximately 475, involving more than 200 companies and 3,900 individual human or animal food products.

The recalls stemmed from public health investigations of a *Salmonella* outbreak that eventually would involve at least 714 confirmed cases of illness in 46 states. According to CDC, related illnesses were determined retrospectively to have begun as early as September 2008, and the outbreak may have contributed to nine deaths. (The CDC noted in its final update in April 2009, that the outbreak was "expected to continue at a low level for the next several months since consumers unaware that they have recalled products in their home continue to consume these products, many of which have a long shelf-life.")

Two months had elapsed between the first recognized cluster of illnesses and the King Nut recall. The CDC on November 10, 2008, had first noticed what it said was a small and highly dispersed multistate cluster of *Salmonella* infections having the same PulseNet "fingerprint" among patients in multiple states. A related cluster of *Salmonella* infections from 17 states was identified by late November. The two investigations were merged in December 2008.

Early efforts to identify the causative food vehicle proved inconclusive; initially chicken was suspected as the source. Peanut butter became the focus after a national case-control study conducted by CDC and public health officials in multiple states in January 2009, which compared foods reported eaten by ill and well persons. Subsequently, the Minnesota Department of Agriculture Laboratory found the outbreak-associated *Salmonella* strain in an opened tub of King Nut peanut butter. At least two other states isolated the same strain in unopened tubs of King Nut peanut butter, which PCA had produced at its plant in Blakely, GA. By mid-January 2009, preliminary studies indicated an association between the *Salmonella* infections and consumption of pre-packaged Austin and Keebler brand peanut butter crackers. The crackers were produced by the Kellogg Company in North Carolina, using peanut paste from PCA.

FDA began an investigation of the Blakely PCA facility on January 9, 2009, which continued until January 27, 2009. This involved sampling and testing, as well as collection of documents deemed necessary to support product recall activities. Environmental sampling (i.e., sampling in the plant rather than the actual product) found two *Salmonella* strains other than the one involved in the outbreak. This investigation also found plant records revealing numerous instances in 2007 and 2008 in which the plant distributed products in commerce even though samples they had submitted to outside testing laboratories had been positive for *Salmonella*. According to FDA, other samples of the product had been resubmitted by the company to other laboratories to obtain a negative result for *Salmonella*.[26]

The PCA recall highlights a number of issues under debate in food safety legislative proposals. Following are examples of these issues.

Registration of Food Facilities

Under current law, FDA requires domestic and foreign food facilities to register once, with no renewal requirement, although they must also report in a timely manner any relevant changes in their registration information.[27] Failure to register is prohibited, but as a practical matter the agency relies on each facility to take that initial step, as well as to report changes. Also, it does not appear that food from unregistered facilities would be considered adulterated or misbranded, and therefore prohibited from being introduced into interstate commerce. (FDA's authority to deem food adulterated or misbranded, and its relationship to "prohibited acts" and associated penalties, is explained in the Appendix.) Exactly how many facilities may fail to register is unknown. In the course of its investigation of PCA, FDA reportedly learned about 20 additional facilities making peanut products without the agency's knowledge.[28] (For example, investigators also found *Salmonella* at a PCA facility in Plainview, TX, that opened in 2005. Texas public health officials had not previously inspected the plant because it had not been registered for a state manufacturer's license.)

Both H.R. 2749 and S. 510 contain provisions to expand federal facility registration requirements, in different ways. Among the key differences, H.R. 2749 would require annual registration renewal and would impose registration fees, while S. 510 would require biennial registration renewal and would not impose registration fees. Both bills would authorize processes by which FDA could suspend a facility's registration. Under H.R. 2749, food products from unregistered facilities (including due to suspension) would be deemed misbranded, so their introduction into interstate commerce would be prohibited. S. 510 would prohibit the importation, the offer to import, and the introduction into interstate commerce of food products from facilities whose registration had been suspended.

The "Attribution Gap"

This incident illustrates that the PulseNet genetic fingerprinting system quickly identified a multistate outbreak caused by a specific strain of *Salmonella*, but that it took about two months of subsequent epidemiologic investigation, including patient interviews, before food vehicles were identified. FDA noted during its investigation that it had not previously considered peanut products to be at high risk of bacterial contamination, but that such products would likely be considered for greater scrutiny in the future.[29]

Food safety officials often lack good information about the kinds of hazards and contaminants that may be present in different kinds of foods. This is particularly true for FDA-regulated foods. Epidemiologic investigation is often needed during outbreak investigation to focus in on suspected food vehicles for testing. This results both in a delay in identifying the contaminated food vehicle (if one is identified at all), and the risk of false attribution, in which investigators erroneously implicate a product based on epidemiologic findings that are later contradicted by laboratory findings.

Economic consequences for producers of the misidentified commodity can be substantial. In addition, a product type may be implicated by the consuming public more broadly than is necessary. (In the case of the peanut products recall, makers of retail peanut butter products reported marked declines in sales of their products, although the products were not found to be contaminated and were not included in the recalls.) As a result, those in the food industry are skeptical about the possible effects of expanding FDA's access to industry food testing results, especially if the parameters governing the agency's disclosure of such information are unclear or subject to agency discretion.

Both H.R. 2749 and S. 510 would require, in somewhat differing ways, that the HHS Secretary work to improve systems of foodborne illness surveillance and outbreak investigation.

Reporting of Food Safety Problems

The FDA Amendments Act of 2007 (FDAAA, P.L. 110-85) added a new section to the FFDCA on reporting requirements, with associated penalties for failure to notify the FDA regarding food safety problems. With certain exceptions, the provision requires persons who register a food facility to report to the FDA within 24 hours after they have determined that an article of food is a "reportable food," defined as a food "for which there is a reasonable probability that the use of, or exposure to, such article of food will cause serious adverse health consequences or death to humans or animals."[30] The requirements were to have been implemented within one year of enactment, or by September 27, 2008. FDA implemented the provision as the Reportable Food Registry in September 2009.[31] Hence, the requirement was not in effect during the PCA outbreak.

It has been argued that PCA would not have been legally required to inform the FDA of the results of testing that found *Salmonella* even if the Reportable Food Registry had been implemented at the time, because the statute leaves the determination of what is reportable up to the registrant.[32] It is unclear whether the company would have had an obligation to report what it called "presumptive" findings of *Salmonella* if it did not determine that there was a reasonable probability of serious adverse health consequences or death associated with the consumption of its products.

H.R. 2749 would amend the authority for the Reportable Food Registry to explicitly require companies to report test results on reportable food products and facilities to the HHS Secretary. In addition, the bill would require reporting by high-risk facilities of test results on finished products if these tests reveal contaminants posing a risk of severe adverse health consequences or death. The bill also would expand the scope of those who now must report foods (i.e., those who must register facilities) to also include farms where food is produced for sale or distribution in interstate commerce, restaurants and other retailers, and those who would be newly required under the bill to register as importers. S. 510 would not amend current law regarding the reporting requirements established by FDAAA.

Access to Records

The FFDCA (as amended by P.L. 107-188, the Public Health Security and Bioterrorism Preparedness and Response Act of 2002) authorizes FDA to require food facilities (but not farms or restaurants) to maintain certain records including immediate prior sources and immediate subsequent recipients. FDA also must be able to inspect and copy records, upon written notice, when the Secretary of HHS has "a reasonable belief that an article of food is adulterated and presents a threat of serious adverse health consequences or death to humans or animals."[33] Some have argued that this authority, which does not appear to provide officials with the ability to access records under other conditions, enabled PCA to hide its problems from regulators. Even where existing authority could be exercised, needed records are not always in an electronic format and/or can be time-consuming and resource-intensive to access during a quickly unfolding investigation. Food safety experts and regulators generally agree that good records, and the ability to access them quickly, are important in traceback investigations in order to quickly determine the cause and source of a problem. But others assert that this must be balanced carefully with industry cost burdens and with commercial privacy concerns.

H.R. 2749 and S. 510 each include provisions, which differ somewhat, that would expand both the HHS Secretary's access to a facility's records and the ability to trace products in the event of a foodborne illness outbreak. In general, H.R. 2749 would appear to allow the Secretary to have routine access to records, no longer requiring that there be any food safety problem triggering such access. S. 510 would retain a trigger, but would lower the threshold for it from the current requirement in two ways; the Secretary would no longer need to believe a product to be adulterated, and would be able to access records for products believed to be affected in a similar manner to products believed to be causing serious health consequences. For example, similar products made by other companies, or products using the same ingredients, could be included in the access authority if the products of one company were linked to an outbreak of illness.

Frequency of Inspections

The FFDCA appears to authorize, but not require, FDA to inspect food facilities; therefore, no inspection frequency is specified. The Blakely, GA, PCA plant had never been inspected by FDA, although the agency had a contract with the Georgia Department of Agriculture to conduct inspections. (See "Role of States and Other "Third Party" Inspectors", below.) Infrequent inspection is not uncommon. The HHS Inspector General recently reported that on average, FDA inspects less than a quarter of food facilities each year, and that 56% of facilities have gone five or more years without an FDA inspection.[34] Whether one or more routine visits by the FDA might have uncovered safety problems at the Blakely plant is unclear. At issue is the frequency and intensity of inspections that would be effective in deterring unsafe conditions and practices; which facilities, if any, should come under greater scrutiny; and what level of funding would be needed to meet the inspection frequency requirements of various proposals.

Both H.R. 2749 and S. 510 would amend FDA's current authority regarding food facility inspections, in a number of ways that differ between the bills. Among other things, the bills address the frequency with which FDA would be required to inspect facilities. H.R. 2749 would require FDA to inspect high-risk facilities every 6 to 12 months, lower-risk facilities every 18 months to three years, and facilities that hold food at least every five years. S. 510 would require FDA to inspect high-risk facilities annually, and non-high-risk facilities at least every four years.

Role of States and Other "Third Party" Inspectors

FDA's resource limitations are one reason the agency relies on states to conduct many safety inspections, as was the case with PCA.[35] Georgia state inspectors had issued numerous citations for unsanitary conditions in the three years prior to the outbreak, but some observers argue that an FDA inspection would have been more rigorous and/or led to sanctions that might have kept unsafe peanut products off the market. The president and CEO of the Kellogg Company told a House panel in early 2009 that food companies commonly rely on third-party private auditors to conduct safety inspections and testing in plants from which they buy ingredients or finished food products. He added that his company utilizes 3,000 ingredients from 1,000 suppliers in its products, that PCA had provided Kellogg with a report of a high safety rating from a widely used industry auditor (AIB International), and that PCA also provided its corporate customers with certificates from private laboratories it had paid to test its products, saying that the products were free of *Salmonella*.[36]

Both H.R. 2749 and S. 510 contain provisions aimed at setting common standards for accrediting third-party auditors and ensuring that they are free of conflicts of interest. Both bills would authorize or require third-party certification of specified entities as a condition to meet certain other requirements in the bills, although the bills vary in how such programs would be implemented.

Hazard Prevention Plans

Unlike USDA-inspected meat and poultry establishments, most FDA-regulated facilities are not required to write and follow plans that analyze potential hazards, implement controls to prevent them, and document compliance. (The agency does require such plans for seafood, low-acid canned foods, and juices, but the programs are not viewed to be as strict as the USDA program.) It has been argued that even when state inspectors visited the Blakely, GA, PCA plant, they were only inspecting conditions on a given day, seeing a "snapshot" that did not necessarily reflect routine conditions. Proponents of hazard prevention planning and documentation argue that regulators could get a better sense of routine conditions if there were records for review documenting a facility's implementation of and ongoing adherence to a hazard prevention plan.

Although they differ in details, both H.R. 2749 and S. 510 would mandate that facilities develop such plans, provide for FDA to set minimum safety standards for the plans, and allow modifications to mitigate regulatory impacts on small businesses.

Melamine Contamination of Animal Feeds (2007) and Dairy Products (2008)[37]

Overview

On March 15, 2007, Menu Foods, a pet food manufacturer, alerted FDA that 13 cats and a dog had died during routine taste trials at the company, reportedly from kidney failure after eating certain cat and dog foods produced at its facilities in Emporia, KS, between December 3, 2006, and March 6, 2007. Consumers and veterinarians in subsequent months reported many more illnesses and deaths of pets potentially associated with a wide variety of pet food brands. As a result, starting on March 16, 2007, more than 150 brands of pet food were voluntarily recalled by a number of companies.

In an investigation, FDA laboratories found melamine and cyanuric acid (a related contaminant linked to the illnesses) in samples of pet food. Cornell University scientists also found melamine in the urine and kidneys of deceased cats that were part of the Menu Foods taste trials. Melamine-tainted ingredients subsequently were found in some hog, chicken, and fish feed. Also, FDA and USDA discovered that some animals that had been fed contaminated feed were processed into food for humans, although they asserted that this presented a very low risk to human health.

Melamine and related compounds have a number of industrial uses, including as an industrial binding agent, flame retardant, and in the manufacture of cooking utensils and plates. The compounds have no approved use as an ingredient in either animal or human food in the United States. If ingested, melamine can crystallize and cause kidney stones and, ultimately, kidney failure, which apparently occurred in the many dog and cat deaths.

FDA traced the melamine to products labeled as wheat gluten and rice protein concentrate imported from China. By February 2008, FDA announced that two Chinese nationals and their businesses, along with a U.S. company and its two top officials, were indicted on federal charges related to importing these products.

Nonetheless, melamine was again found in a number of Chinese-sourced human foods later the same year. On November 12, 2008, FDA issued an import alert for all milk products, milk-derived ingredients, and finished food products containing milk if they are from China. The alert stated that these products could be contaminated by melamine or cyanuric acid. FDA explained that in September 2008, it had become aware of reports that more than 53,000 infants in China had been sickened, including 13,000 who were hospitalized and four who had died, due to consumption of infant formula tainted with melamine.[38] Milk used in the formula was implicated as the source of the melamine, which was added to watered-down bulk milk at collection points in China to inflate the protein content. This "economic adulteration" also apparently was the reason melamine had found its way into pet foods and animal feed ingredients.[39]

The import alert for milk products was added to existing alerts for Chinese-sourced vegetable protein products and animal foods. Under the alerts, which remain in effect, these products cannot be imported from China unless they have been shown, through independent (third-party) laboratory testing, to be free of melamine or cyanuric acid.[40] An importing firm can request exemption from these requirements—which can greatly slow if not completely stop its imports—by demonstrating that it has adequate safety controls in place and that it has had five consecutive non-violative shipments.[41]

Chinese government sources also indicated that contaminated milk components, especially milk powder, were used in a variety of finished foods dispersed throughout the Chinese food supply chain. More than a dozen countries throughout Asia and Europe, along with Australia and the United States, soon reported that they had detected contamination of milk-derived ingredients and products with melamine or cyanuric acid. These products included candy and beverages found in the United States by the FDA. In other countries, melamine was detected in Chinese-sourced fluid and powdered milk, yogurt, frozen desserts, biscuits, cakes and cookies, soft candy products, chocolates, and beverages.

In a health information advisory issued on September 12, 2008, FDA had stated that there was no known threat of contamination in infant formulas "that have met the requirements to sell such products in the United States." FDA said that it had been reassured by companies that manufacture infant formula for the U.S. market that they are not importing formula or sourcing milk-based materials from China.[42] Nonetheless, China was exporting dairy proteins and other products to the United States for some time, but at somewhat low levels, according to USDA trade data. China accounted for no more than 2% of all U.S. imports of casein (a dairy protein) from January 2007 through July 2008. According to a U.S. government study, two-thirds of all casein purchases in 2002 were used here for nondairy food products, primarily imitation cheese and coffee creamers.[43]

The melamine contamination incidents highlight a number of issues under debate in food safety legislative proposals. Following are examples of these issues.

Confluence of the Food Supply for Humans and Other Animals

The melamine incident illustrates the confluence of ingredients (whether legal or illegal) found in both animal and human foods. The initial U.S. investigation had focused on melamine-contaminated pet foods. It was soon found that the same ingredients were used to manufacture feeds for food animals. For example, it was reported that Tyson foods processed hogs for food that had been fed melamine-contaminated feed.[44] As has been reported, melamine in animal feed not only was transferred to and detected in human foods (for example, it was being detected in eggs in China), it also was being added directly to milk used for infant formula and other dairy products intended for human use.

The FFDCA defines "food" as "(1) articles used for food or drink for man or other animals, (2) chewing gum, and (3) articles used for components of any such article,"[45] effectively charging the agency to regulate both human and animal foods with equal diligence. FDA's authorities over animal food and feeds would not be diminished under the pending food safety bills.

Reporting of Food Safety Problems

Some observers noted that the contaminated pet food incident involved a long delay between when the Menu Foods company first learned of the deaths among its taste-trial animals and when it notified FDA and product recipients of the problem.[46] The incident also showed the weakness in foodborne illness recognition and reporting by veterinarians and others caring for sick dogs and cats, for which there is no national system comparable to that for reporting of foodborne illnesses in humans.

It was in large part as a result of the melamine pet food incident that Congress, in the FDA Amendments Act of 2007 (FDAAA, P.L. 110-85), established the reporting requirements discussed earlier in this report. (See "Reporting of Food Safety Problems" in the earlier section regarding the peanut products recall.) As such, the requirements were not in effect during the pet food incident. However, had the requirements been in effect, the responsible companies might not have been required to report for a number of reasons, such as a firm's interpretation of the reporting trigger "reasonable probability."[47]

As discussed earlier, the reporting requirements established by FDAAA define a reportable food as a food "for which there is a reasonable probability that the use of, or exposure to, such article of food will cause serious adverse health consequences or death to humans *or animals.*" (Emphasis added.) Consequently, had the reporting provision been in force at the time, the Menu Foods company would not have been freed of the obligation to report solely because the problem involved pet food. The language for the reporting requirement is in keeping with the common definition of "food" in the FFDCA, noted earlier as food for "man or other animals," and is consistent with the frequent confluence of the two food supplies.

Authority to Recall Products

The melamine incidents also focused attention on the FDA's authorities and procedures for recalling foods.[48] An August 2009 report by the HHS Office of Inspector General (OIG) found, for example, that the FDA's lack of statutory authority to order a recall (or to assess penalties for recall violations) was only one reason the agency encountered difficulty in ensuring that the contaminated pet food was quickly taken off the market. The OIG also uncovered other contributing factors, including the agency's failure to closely follow its own recall policies or to adequately determine the effectiveness of the recall, which the agency could have accomplished without new authorities. Among the OIG's recommendations were to establish mandatory industry recall requirements including a written strategy, prompt effectiveness checks, and periodic status reports.[49]

Both H.R. 2749 and S. 510 would grant FDA the authority to mandate recalls to address food safety problems. The bills propose somewhat different approaches regarding the triggers allowing or requiring a mandatory recall, the conditions and processes by which a recall mandate may be appealed, requirements regarding notification of recipients of affected products and of the public, and other particulars.

Oversight of Import Safety

The melamine incidents also illustrate the challenges of ensuring the safety of imported foods and food ingredients, which have increased significantly over the past several decades to about 15% of the food consumed here. (For some products such as seafood the proportion is far higher.) In the case of wheat gluten, to which the melamine was added, the United States imports almost all of its supply. A frequently quoted statistic is that FDA only physically inspects or tests samples of approximately 1% of all food import "lines."[50] Even if FDA were given a clear mandate to inspect foreign facilities that export to the United States, there are an estimated 200,000 of them (and likely many more that are not registered), which the FDA now rarely enters.

H.R. 2749 and S. 510 would make a number of changes to FDA's authority regarding imported foods, including requiring U.S. importers of foreign foods to implement good importer practices, essentially a set of standards to ensure the products (and their sources) meet minimum safety requirements; requiring third party certification of certain higher-risk food imports; developing agreements with foreign countries whereby U.S. authorities determine that their safety systems meet or exceed U.S. standards, at least for certain designated products; and placing more FDA assets in foreign countries to conduct inspections or assist foreign regulators, particularly for those countries that are the largest source of imports.

E. coli O157:H7 Outbreak from Spinach (2006)[51]

Overview

In September 2006, CDC began receiving reports of clusters of patients with confirmed cases of *E. coli* O157:H7 infection, linked through the PulseNet system, which would soon be recognized as a single foodborne illness outbreak with more than 200 confirmed illnesses. Twenty-six states reported cases. Three persons died, and more than 100 were hospitalized, nearly a third of them with hemolytic-uremic syndrome (HUS), a life-threatening complication associated with *E. coli* O157:H7 infections.

Epidemiological investigation, based on food history surveys of persons with illness compared with control subjects, pointed to fresh spinach as a possible source of infection. Based on this epidemiological evidence, on September 14, 2006, FDA issued a nationwide alert advising consumers to avoid eating any brand of packaged fresh spinach. The progressing investigation revealed that the illnesses were most often associated with Dole brand baby spinach processed by a facility in San Juan Bautista, CA, owned by Natural Selection Foods (NSF) and doing business as Earthbound Farm. After discussions with FDA and California public health officials, NSF on September 15, 2006, initiated a national recall of all brands of all products they packed that contained spinach and that had "best if used by" dates between August 17 and October 1 of that year. On September 20, 2006, almost a week after FDA's first consumer advisory was issued, investigators made the first laboratory identification of the outbreak *E. coli* strain in a bag of Dole baby spinach.

Although the outbreak strain of *E. coli* was subsequently found in a number of packaged spinach products, investigators were unable to find the pathogen in samples taken at the processor or to identify how the pathogen could have been introduced there. During product traceback activities using product codes from bags of the implicated spinach, investigators sampled four specific farm fields in Monterey and San Benito Counties, CA. Sampling revealed *E. coli* O157:H7 in each of the four fields, but only one of the fields and its surrounds had the outbreak strain of the pathogen. For this field, the outbreak strain was found in river water, cattle feces, and wild pig feces, the closest a mile from the spinach field. The field was part of a large ranch where the land was primarily used for cattle grazing, with only a small portion used for ready-to-eat crop production. Although investigators found evidence of wild pigs around both the cattle pastures and crop-growing regions of the ranch, no definitive determination was made regarding how the pathogen contaminated the spinach.

The *E. coli* O157:H7 outbreak due to contaminated fresh spinach highlights several issues under debate in food safety legislative proposals. Following are examples of these issues.

Foodborne Illness Surveillance and Outbreak Investigation

In 2006 testimony before a Senate committee, a CDC official observed

> The [spinach] event illustrates how a large and widespread outbreak can occur, appearing first as small clusters, and then rapidly increasing if a popular commercial product is contaminated. It also illustrates the importance of existing public health networks: the laboratories performing PulseNet "fingerprinting"; the epidemiologists interviewing patients and healthy people and collecting leftover spinach; the multi-disciplinary approach to the investigation; and the close communication and collaboration among local, state, and federal officials. This investigation illustrates what a robust public health system can do and lays down a benchmark for the future. Without question, a rapid and accurate analysis of and response to an outbreak will result in prevention of exposure to contaminated products and will stop further illness and death.[52]

As this statement and the discussion at the beginning of this memorandum suggest, foodborne illness surveillance and outbreak response have progressed significantly in the past decade, but many limitations remain.

Both H.R. 2749 and S. 510 would require, in somewhat different ways, that the HHS Secretary work to improve systems of foodborne illness surveillance and outbreak investigation, information sharing and coordination among public health officials, and incorporation of research findings into foodborne illness prevention and outbreak response activities.

Determining and Ranking Risk

Almost all food safety experts agree on the need to concentrate finite resources on the highest-risk products, processes, and operations, and that the decisions on what these are must be based on authoritative information supported by sound science. However, achieving this goal can be difficult, particularly given the constantly evolving ways in which food is produced, distributed and consumed. For example, public attention through much of the 1990s focused on outbreaks of *E. coli* infections associated with the consumption of undercooked or otherwise mishandled hamburger meat, as the pathogen is sometimes found in animal intestines and feces. However, as public health officials acknowledge, outbreaks associated with the consumption of fresh produce have become more common in recent years. Spinach in particular had not been identified as a source of *E. coli* O157:H7 outbreaks before the 2006 incident, but other leafy greens were implicated in a number of outbreaks, several of them traced to California.[53] Consumers have responded to dietary advice that they consume more fresh produce, and are buying and consuming it in pre-washed and packaged forms that generally were not available 20 years ago. These types of products are most frequently mass-produced in centralized locations and then shipped to many distributors nationally. As a result, contamination on a single farm can result in illnesses across the country. Like the food system itself, assessments of food safety hazards, and how to address them, will have to evolve continually as well.

Determining the food safety risks associated with specific foods or practices underlies a number of provisions in H.R. 2749 and S. 510. For example, both bills would require the HHS Secretary to review relevant health, epidemiologic and other data every two years to identify the most significant foodborne contaminants, and apply such information (in somewhat different ways) when issuing standards, guidance, and/or regulations. Both bills imply that the Secretary would have to determine relative risks before issuing standards for safe produce, setting any required certifications for certain types of imported foods, or ranking which food facilities should be inspected the most frequently. In the case of inspection frequencies, for example, H.R. 2749 states that the Secretary, if altering inspection frequencies, must consider the type of food, the facility's compliance history, and other factors that are, essentially, determinants of risk.

On-Farm Food Safety Standards

Many food safety advocates and public health officials and a number of produce industry leaders agree that produce-related outbreaks are a growing challenge. Many are calling for the development of more stringent FDA-issued and enforced standards for on-farm production where, it is believed, many of the pathogens causing these outbreaks can originate.

Nonetheless, not everyone is convinced that mandatory standards are necessary. A number of opponents support the generally voluntary approach taken by FDA through the issuance of nonbinding guidance documents for producers and others who handle fresh produce. They may also support recent produce industry efforts to self-impose standards through binding marketing arrangements, which they believe may generate more enthusiastic support and participation among producers than would the imposition of a government-enforced approach. Under the Agricultural Marketing Act of 1946,[54] USDA's Agricultural Marketing Service (AMS) has implemented a wide range of these voluntary testing and process verification programs. Funded by industry user fees, these services use independent, third-party audits and other standardized procedures to help producers certify that products meet buyer specifications. Although some of these programs can be, and are, designed to ensure the safety of certain food commodities from a public health standpoint, they are not regulatory by nature. Rather, they are intended to facilitate commercial agreements in the trade or to provide consumers with more information about their prospective purchases.[55] AMS recently proposed a marketing agreement for leafy green vegetables.[56]

Moreover, it is argued that producers should not be required to take on new responsibilities until more is known about exactly what types of interventions are needed and effective. Others have argued that while there may be gaps in the knowledge base, enough is known to address some of the more obvious practices, such as basic worker sanitation, the separation of animals and their waste from produce fields, use of clean water, and so forth. As noted above, the definitive cause of the contamination of spinach, leading to the nationwide outbreak, was never established. As a CDC official observed, "As this and other outbreaks indicate, research should focus on tracing the specific pathways that connect fields of leafy green vegetables with potential animal reservoirs of *E. coli* and other disease-causing microbes."[57]

H.R. 2749 and S. 510 would require, in somewhat different ways, that the HHS Secretary (i.e., FDA) develop safety standards for raw fruits and vegetables, primarily those for which the Secretary (FDA) has determined there is a need to reduce the risk of serious illness or death.[58]

Appendix. Key Definitions and Authorities in the FFDCA Regarding Food[59]

Adulteration: The FFDCA has multiple definitions of adulteration that differ, depending on whether they apply to food, drugs, or other products. With respect to the general safety of food, adulteration is defined in FFDCA § 402(a) [21 USC § 342(a)], as follows:

A food shall be deemed to be adulterated—
(1) If it bears or contains any poisonous or deleterious substance which may render it injurious to health; but in case the substance is not an added substance such food shall not be considered adulterated under this clause if the quantity of such substance in such food does not ordinarily render it injurious to health; [or]
(2)(A) if it bears or contains any added poisonous or added deleterious substance (other than a substance that is a pesticide chemical residue in or on a raw agricultural commodity or processed food, a food additive, a color additive, or a new animal drug) that is unsafe within the meaning of section 406; or (B) if it bears or contains a pesticide chemical residue that is unsafe within the meaning of section 408(a); or (C) if it is or if it bears or contains (i) any food additive that is unsafe within the meaning of section 409; or (ii) a new animal drug (or conversion product thereof) that is unsafe within the meaning of section 512; or
(3) if it consists in whole or in part of any filthy, putrid, or decomposed substance, or if it is otherwise unfit for food; or
(4) if it has been prepared, packed, or held under insanitary conditions whereby it may have become contaminated with filth, or whereby it may have been rendered injurious to health; or
(5) if it is, in whole or in part, the product of a diseased animal or of an animal which has died otherwise than by slaughter; or

(6) if its container is composed, in whole or in part, of any poisonous or deleterious substance which may render the contents injurious to health; or

(7) if it has been intentionally subjected to radiation, unless the use of the radiation was in conformity with a regulation or exemption in effect pursuant to section 409.

Additional subsections of § 402 define several additional specific types of adulteration, or adulteration of specific types of foods. *FFDCA § 301(a) - (c) provide that introducing adulterated food into commerce, adulterating food that is in commerce, or the receipt and delivery of adulterated food in commerce is prohibited.* See the definition of "Prohibited Acts," below.

Facility: FFDCA § 415(b) [21 USC § 350d(b)] defines a food facility as "any factory, warehouse, or establishment (including a factory, warehouse, or establishment of an importer) that manufactures, processes, packs, or holds food. Such term does not include farms; restaurants; other retail food establishments; nonprofit food establishments in which food is prepared for or served directly to the consumer; or fishing vessels (except such vessels engaged in processing as defined in section 123.3(k) of title 21, Code of Federal Regulations)."

The term "facility" is only defined for the purposes of FFDCA § 415 and not for the entirety of the FFDCA. FFDCA § 415(a)(1) states that "The Secretary shall by regulation require that any facility engaged in manufacturing, processing, packing, or holding food for consumption in the United States be registered with the Secretary. To be registered—(A) for a domestic facility, the owner, operator, or agent in charge of the facility shall submit a registration to the Secretary; and (B) for a foreign facility, the owner, operator, or agent in charge of the facility shall submit a registration to the Secretary and shall include with the registration the name of the United States agent for the facility."

Food: FFDCA § 201(f) [21 USC § 321(f)] defines food as "(1) articles used for food or drink for man or other animals, (2) chewing gum, and (3) articles used for components of any such article." *Unless a provision in law regarding food limits its applicability to one or the other, it would apply equally to both human foods, and to animal foods and feeds.*

Misbranding: FFDCA § 403 [21 USC § 343] defines a number of conditions under which a food would be deemed to be misbranded, beginning with a broad provision in paragraph (a) saying that a food is deemed misbranded if its label "is false or misleading in any particular." Similar to the definition of adulteration, numerous specific types of misbranding are also defined. *FFDCA § 301(a) - (c) provide that introducing misbranded food into commerce, misbranding food that is in commerce, or the receipt and delivery of misbranded food in commerce is prohibited.* See the definition of "Prohibited Acts," below.

Person: FFDCA § 201(e) [21 USC § 321(e)] defines "person" to include an individual, partnership, corporation, and association.

Prohibited Acts: Acts that are stated to be prohibited are added to a list of "prohibited acts" in FFDCA § 301 [21 USC § 331]. As described earlier, along with many other listed prohibited acts in FFDCA § 301, *paragraphs (a) through (c) provide that introducing adulterated or misbranded food into commerce; adulterating or misbranding food that is in commerce; or the receipt and delivery of adulterated or misbranded food in commerce is prohibited.* Pursuant to FFDCA § 303 [21 USC § 333], in general, any person who violates a provision of FFDCA § 301 may be subject to civil or criminal penalties, including imprisonment, fines, or both. The criminal penalties provisions provided for in the FFDCA are adjusted by 18 U.S.C. §§ 3559 and 3571. Additional sanctions may apply for drugs or devices, and certain exceptions may be made, including for the misbranding of foods.

End Notes

[1] U.S. Government Accountability Office, *High-Risk Series: An Update*, GAO-09-271, January 2009, pp. 71-72, http://www.gao.gov/new.items/d09271.pdf, and related food safety reports and testimony.

[2] For more information on the roles of FDA, FSIS, and other federal agencies in the nation's food safety efforts, see CRS Report RS22600, *The Federal Food Safety System: A Primer*, by Geoffrey S. Becker (in particular Tables 1 and 2). See also CRS Report RL34334, *The Food and Drug Administration: Budget and Statutory History, FY1980-FY2007*, coordinated by Judith A. Johnson.

[3] Paul S. Mead et al., "Food-Related Illness and Death in the United States," *Emerging Infectious Diseases*, vol. 5, pp. 607-625, 1999 (hereafter Mead article), http://www.cdc.gov/ncidod/EID/vol5no5/mead.htm. These estimates were derived from a variety of sources. See also, CDC, "Foodborne Illness: Frequently Asked Questions," http://www.cdc.gov/foodsafety/.

[4] In the United States, states may mandate that laboratories, health care providers, and others report cases of illness to state authorities. Reporting by states to the Centers for Disease Control and Prevention (CDC) is voluntary.

[5] Mead article. See also CDC, "Foodborne Illness: Frequently Asked Questions," http://www.cdc.gov/foodsafety/.

[6] For information about foodborne illness monitoring programs in general, see CDC, "Overview of CDC Food Safety Activities and Programs," http://www.cdc.gov/foodsafety/fsactivities.htm.

[7] CDC, "FoodNet–Foodborne Diseases Active Surveillance Network," http://www.cdc.gov/foodnet/. The 10 FoodNet sites—the states of Connecticut, Georgia, Maryland, Minnesota, New Mexico, Tennessee, and Oregon, and certain counties in California, Colorado, and New York—are the sites for CDC's Emerging Infections Program. They were selected to be generally representative of the U.S. population. FoodNet surveillance in these sites captures a range of regional and ethnic experiences with foodborne illness.

[8] However, additional studies based on FoodNet-identified cases of illness can establish attribution to food vehicles.

[9] CDC, "Preliminary FoodNet Data on the Incidence of Infection with Pathogens Transmitted Commonly Through Food–10 States, 2008," MMWR, vol. 58, no. 13 (April 10, 2009), pp. 333-337. "Healthy People 2010" is a set of national health objectives developed by governmental and nongovernmental scientists identifying the most significant preventable threats to health and establishing national goals to reduce them. Food safety is one of 28 focus areas. See http://www.healthypeople.gov/.

[10] CDC, "Q&A for the FoodNet MMWR with data from 2009," April 13, 2010, p. 1, http://www.cdc.gov/foodnet/ mmwr/2010_FoodNet_MMWR_QA.pdf.

[11] CDC, "OutbreakNet Team Overview," http://www.cdc.gov/foodborneoutbreaks/.

[12] Refer also to footnote 5, regarding the fact that some proportion of foodborne illness results from causes (etiologies) that have not yet been identified.

[13] Center for Science in the Public Interest, "Outbreak Alert! 2008," December, 2008, http://cspinet.org/new/pdf/ outbreak_alert_2008_report_final.pdf. This report describes a subset of FBDOs that have been attributed to specific foods.

[14] Michael Lynch et al., "Surveillance for Foodborne-Disease Outbreaks–United States, 1998-2002," MMWR Surveillance Summaries, vol. 55(SS10) (November 10, 2006), pp. 1-34.

[15] CDC PulseNet program, http://www.cdc.gov/pulsenet/.

[16] FSIS conducts routine Salmonella testing of meat and poultry products, and inputs genetic "fingerprints" from a subset of these samples into the PulseNet database. This is the most comprehensive public-sector sampling program for bacterial foodborne pathogens.

[17] Portions of this discussion are drawn from CRS Report RL34167, The FDA's Authority to Recall Products, by Vanessa K. Burrows, where additional information, including arguments for and against mandatory recall authority, may be found.

[18] U.S. Government Accountability Office, Food Safety: Actions Needed by USDA and FDA to Ensure that Companies Promptly Carry Out Recalls, GAO-RCED-00-195, August 2000, pp. 15-16 and 37-38, http://www.gao.gov/. The agency was called the General Accounting Office at the time of publication.

[19] 21 C.F.R. § 7.3(g). The definition of a recall "does not include a market withdrawal or a stock recovery," which are defined in the regulation.

[20] 21 C.F.R. § 7.3(m)(1) through (3).

[21] FDA, "Recalls, Market Withdrawals, and Safety Alerts," http://www.fda.gov/safety/recalls/default.htm.

[22] FDA, "Enforcement Reports," http://www.fda.gov/Safety/ Recalls/EnforcementReports/default.htm.

[23] For more information on meat and poultry recall authority, see CRS Report RL34313, *The USDA's Authority to Recall Meat and Poultry Products*, by Cynthia Brougher and Geoffrey S. Becker.

[24] Generally, this trend also applies if data for FY2009 are excluded.

[25] Unless otherwise noted, information for this section is derived from CDC, "Investigation Update: Outbreak of *Salmonella* Typhimurium Infections, 2008–2009" (final web update of the investigation), April 29, 2009, http://www.cdc.gov/salmonella/typhimurium/update.html; FDA, "Peanut Products Recall," http://www.fda.gov/Safety/ Recalls/MajorProductRecalls/Peanut/default.htm; and testimony of Stephen F. Sundlof, Director, FDA Center for Food Safety and Applied Nutrition, hearing of the House Committee on Energy and Commerce, Subcommittee on Oversight and Investigations, *Foodborne Illness Outbreak Associated with Salmonella*, 111th Cong., 1st sess., February 11, 2009.

[26] The FDA "Form 483" inspectional observation reports, which contain these findings, were accessed on September 10, 2009, at http://www.fda.gov/AboutFDA/CentersOffices/ORA/ORAElectronicReadingRoom/ucm109818.htm.

[27] This requirement was enacted as a new Sec. 415 of the FFDCA by P.L. 107-188, the Public Health Security and Bioterrorism Preparedness and Response Act of 2002.

[28] See for example "FDA Hasn't Intensified Inspections at Peanut Facilities, Despite Illness," *The Washington Post*, April 2, 2009.

[29] According to FDA, "The term 'High Risk Foods' is used to denote foods that may present hazards, which FDA believes, may present a high potential to cause harm from their consumption. The firms that produce high risk foods have priority for inspectional purposes." FDA, Compliance Program Guide 7303.803, "Domestic Food Safety Program," Part II, p. 1, November 2008. http://www.fda.gov/Food/GuidanceComplianceRegulatoryInformation/ComplianceEnforcement/ucm071496.htm.

[30] FFDCA § 417; 21 U.S.C. 350f.

[31] FDA, "Reportable Food Registry," http://www.fda.gov/food/foodsafety/foodsafetyprograms/rfr/default.htm.

[32] See CRS Report R40450, *Penalties Under the Federal Food, Drug, and Cosmetic Act (FFDCA) That May Pertain to Adulterated Peanut Products*, by Vanessa K. Burrows and Brian T. Yeh, where this argument is explained on page 4.

[33] FFDCA, § 414; 21 U.S.C. § 350(c).

[34] HHS, Office of Inspector General, *FDA Inspections of Domestic Food Facilities*, Report OEI-02-08-00080, p. ii, April 2010, http://oig.hhs.gov/oei/reports/oei-02-08-00080.pdf.

[35] The lack of sufficient funding and staff to meet FDA's responsibilities was the key theme of a late 2007 report by an FDA scientific advisory panel. See "Paying for Food Safety" in CRS Report R40443, *Food Safety: Selected Issues and Bills in the 111th Congress*, by Geoffrey S. Becker, for more information on food safety funding issues.

[36] Testimony and comments of A. D. David Mackay, President and Chief Executive Officer, Kellogg Company, hearing on *The Salmonella Outbreak: The Role of Industry in Protecting the Nation's Food Supply*, before the House Energy and Commerce Subcommittee on Oversight and Investigations, March 19, 2009.

[37] Unless otherwise noted, information for this section is derived from information on the FDA website and material prepared previously by CRS, including CRS Report RL34198, *U.S. Food and Agricultural Imports: Safeguards and Selected Issues*, by Geoffrey S. Becker.

[38] The Chinese as of early 2009 revised these numbers upward, to an official count of seven infant deaths and 300,000 illnesses due to consumption of melamine-tainted milk products.

[39] The FFDCA states that a food shall be deemed adulterated if, among other things, "any substance has been added thereto or mixed or packed therewith so as to increase its bulk or weight, or reduce its quality or strength, or make it appear better or of greater value than it

is." FFDCA § 402(b)(4); 21 U.S.C. § 342(b)(4). This so-called economic adulteration is intentional, although the intent is typically to defraud, not to cause harm. The melamine incident showed that harm is, however, a possible consequence.

[40] FDA Import Alert #99-30 (for milk products) and other alerts regarding melamine are available at FDA, "Import Alerts," http://www.fda.gov/ForIndustry/ImportProgram/ImportAlerts/default.htm, by searching for alerts involving products imported from China.

[41] FDA announced in early 2009 that it planned to begin testing aquaculture imports from China for melamine. Studies have shown that fish can retain high levels of melamine after receiving feed contaminated with it. Earlier, in December 2008, FSIS said that as a precautionary measure it had begun 12 weeks of sampling to test meat, poultry and dairy products for melamine. No problems were reported.

[42] On November 26, 2008, the Associated Press (AP) reported that the FDA had found traces of melamine in samples of U.S. infant formula. FDA officials reportedly told the AP that the trace amounts had occurred during manufacturing, not intentionally, and posed no health concerns. On November 28, 2008, FDA reported, "To date, FDA tests have found extremely low levels of melamine in one infant formula sample and extremely low levels of cyanuric acid in another. The levels were so low (well below 1 ppm) that they do not pose a health risk to infants." http://www.fda.gov/NewsEvents/PublicHealthFocus/ucm179005.htm.

[43] U.S. International Trade Commission, *Conditions of Competition for Milk Protein Products in the U.S. Market* (Investigation No. 332—453), May 2004.

[44] See for example "U.S. Has Its Own Melamine Problem," *The Seattle Post-Intelligencer*, November 26, 2008.

[45] FFDCA § 201(f); 21 USC § 321(f).

[46] See for example U.S. Congress, Senate Committee on Appropriations, Subcommittee on Labor, Health and Human Services, Education, and Related Agencies, *Hearing toExamine the Current Pet Food Recall*, 110th Cong., 1st sess., April 12, 2007, S.Hrg. 110-72 (Washington: GPO, 2007).

[47] Portions of this discussion are taken from CRS Report R40450, *Penalties Under the Federal Food, Drug, and Cosmetic Act (FFDCA) That May Pertain to Adulterated Peanut Products*, by Vanessa K. Burrows and Brian T. Yeh.

[48] Although FDA publishes guidance for industry on how to carry out a food product recall, the agency's current authority to mandate a food product recall is limited to infant formula. See CRS Report RL34167, *The FDA's Authority to Recall Products*, by Vanessa K. Burrows.

[49] HHS, OIG, *Review of the Food and Drug Administration's Monitoring of Pet Food Recalls*, August 12, 2009, http://oig.hhs.gov/oas/reports/region1/10701503.asp. See also Jennifer C. Smith, "Food Safety Groups: FDA Should Act Now on OIG Recommendations," *FDA Week*, August 28, 2009.

[50] A "line" is a portion of an import shipment that is listed separately on that import's entry document. An item in a shipment must have a separate line if its tariff description differs from other items in that shipment. Lines have no standard size, so the 1% is not a measurement of volume. For more information, including a source for this estimate, see CRS Report RL34198, *U.S. Food and Agricultural Imports: Safeguards and Selected Issues*, by Geoffrey S. Becker.

[51] Unless otherwise noted, information for this section is derived from archived CRS Report RL33722, *Food Safety: Federal and State Response to the Spinach E. coli Outbreak*, by Donna V. Porter; CDC, "Multi-State Outbreak of *E. coli* O157:H7 Infections from Spinach," http://www.cdc.gov/ecoli/2006/september/; FDA, "Spinach and *E. coli* Outbreak," http://www.fda.gov/NewsEvents/PublicHealthFocus/ucm179124.htm; and a series of reports on the outbreak investigation by the California Department of Health Services and the FDA, http://www.dhs.ca.gov/fdb/ HTML/Food/EnvInvRpt.htm.

[52] Statement of Lonnie J. King, CDC Senior Veterinarian, before the Senate Committee on Health, Education, Labor and Pensions, hearing on "Food Safety: Current Challenges and New Ideas to Safeguard Consumers," November 15, 2006, hereafter Statement of Lonnie J. King, November 15, 2006.

[53] Ibid.

[54] 7 U.S.C. § 1621 note.

[55] These marketing arrangements are described in more detail in CRS Report RL34612, *Food Safety on the Farm: Federal Programs and Selected Proposals*, by Geoffrey S. Becker.

[56] USDA, Agricultural Marketing Service, "Leafy Green Vegetables Handled in the United States; Hearing on Proposed Marketing Agreement No. 970," 74 *Federal Register* 45565-45574, September 3, 2009.

[57] Statement of Lonnie J. King, November 15, 2006.

[58] For more information on the specific proposals in each bill, see CRS Report RL34612, *Food Safety on the Farm: Federal Programs and Selected Proposals*, by Geoffrey S. Becker.

[59] A version of the FFDCA is available on FDA's website at http://www.fda.gov/RegulatoryInformation/Legislation/FederalFoodDrugandCosmeticActFDCAct/default.htm.

In: Foodborne Illness, E. coli and Salmonella   ISBN: 978-1-62100-052-5
Editors: M. Laskaris and F. Korol   © 2011 Nova Science Publishers, Inc.

Chapter 2

Food Safety: Federal and State Response to the Spinach E.coli Outbreak

Donna V. Porter and Sarah A. Lister

Abstract

In September 2006, the Food and Drug Administration (FDA) and the Centers for Disease Control and Prevention (CDC) began receiving reports on clusters of patients in various states confirmed to have *E. coli* infections. By early October, 199 people in 26 states had become ill — 102 had been hospitalized, 31 had developed hemolytic uremic syndrome (HUS), a type of kidney failure, and three had died.

Escherichia coli O157:H7 (*E. coli*) is a bacterium found in animal feces that causes diarrhea and abdominal cramps within days of exposure. An infection can lead to HUS and, in some cases, death. Public health laboratories perform a type of DNA fingerprinting to determine whether a sample taken from a patient matches those taken from other patients and contaminated food during an outbreak. The time from exposure to confirmation of an *E. coli* infection can take two to three weeks.

As the number of infections increased, an investigation that included FDA, CDC, and state and local public healthofficials was launched. Starting on September 14 and continuing into early October, FDA and CDC released nearly daily statements on the status of the investigation, alerting the public to the number of cases, states with confirmed cases, spinach product recalls, agency actions, and consumer advice on consumption of spinach products. Investigators were able to trace the outbreak back to several farm fields in the Salinas Valley of California. While the investigation continues, there is evidence that nearby livestock, feral pigs or other environmental sources may have contaminated one or more of the fields.

Since the outbreak, FDA has advised growers of fresh produce that they need to develop and implement voluntary guidelines to prevent outbreaks of food-borne diseases. FDA has also announced that it will convene a public meeting on the issue once the investigation is complete. Several growers groups have called for their industry to use the best agricultural and processing practices to prevent such outbreaks, not least because losses to the industry from the spinach outbreak have been estimated at $100 million.

In October 2006, the House Committee on Energy and Commerce asked FDA to explain its role in detecting contaminated food, particularly in the recent tainted spinach case. The request sought details about the agency's food safety procedures used in emergency situations.

Both proponents and opponents of the National Uniformity for Food Act (S. 3128, H.R. 4167) have weighed in on how it would have affected the *E. coli* outbreak. Opponents believe that states' ability to act would have been compromised, while proponents claim that the legislation would not have affected state adulteration or inspection authorities.

Legislators may address the recent *E. coli* outbreak during reauthorization of the farm bill in the 110th Congress, when the proposal for a single food safety agency with increased powers may be considered.

Introduction

In September 2006, government officials were alerted to an outbreak of *E. coli* O157:H7 infections associated with the consumption of tainted fresh spinach. For several weeks, the Food and Drug Administration (FDA) and the Centers for Disease Control and Prevention (CDC) investigated the situation as additional cases were identified nearly daily. This report details the events as they unfolded, and includes the number of cases, the detection of the first case, and the process by which relevant agencies acted as subsequent cases were reported. This report will be updated in response to any further developments.

Background

The public first became aware of a new deadly strain of *E. coli* in 1982 during an outbreak associated with ground beef. *Escherichia coli* is a bacterium normally found in the intestines of humans and animals. Most strains of *E. coli* are harmless. Several strains, including serotype O157:H7, may cause serious illness in humans, though they are frequently found in livestock feces, particularly in cattle manure. In humans, infection with *E. coli* O157:H7 can cause diarrhea that is often bloody and accompanied by abdominal cramps. Fever may occur. Symptoms usually develop in two to four days, but may emerge as quickly as a day or up to a week after exposure. Healthy adults can generally recover completely from infection within a week. Some individuals, however, especially young children and the elderly, can develop hemolytic uremic syndrome (HUS) as a result of infection. HUS can lead to serious kidney damage and even death. In terms of treatment, antibiotics are not indicated and may be harmful. Due to the severity of illness, treatment of these infections often requires hospitalization. Patients who experience kidney failure may need dialysis. For the remainder of this report, "*E. coli*" will refer to the *E. coli* O157:H7 strain implicated in the spinach outbreak.

The Process of *E. coli* Case Confirmation

The cases of *E. coli* linked to spinach consumption, as discussed in this report, are "confirmed," meaning that victims have been shown, by laboratory analysis of specimens, to be infected with the organism. There are a number of reasons why confirmation may not occur for all victims of an outbreak, though for serious illnesses such as *E. coli*, the proportion of cases that are investigated with laboratory testing is generally higher than with milder foodborne illness. The time from the beginning of a patient's illness to confirmation of whether the patient is part of an outbreak typically takes from two to three weeks. In the case of the *E. coli* outbreak in spinach, the average time for confirmation of cases was about 15 days.[1]

In most cases of *E. coli* infection, public healthlaboratories in states and some cities perform a type of DNA fingerprinting on *E. coli* samples. Investigators determine whether the DNA fingerprinting pattern of the bacterium from one patient is the same as that from other infected patients and from contaminated food. Bacteria with the same DNA fingerprint are likely to have come from the same source.

A series of steps takes place between the point when a patient is infected and the point when public healthofficials can confirm whether the patient is part of an *E. coli*outbreak. As a result, there is generally a two- to three-week delay between the start of the illness and confirmation of the patient's connection to the outbreak.

This series breaks down as follows: In the case of *E. coli*, an incubation period from the time of eating contaminated food to the beginning of the first symptoms is typically two to four days. The time from the first symptom until the person seeks medical care, when a diarrhea sample is collected for testing, is generally one to five days. The process of laboratory diagnosis, which begins when a patient provides a sample and *E. coli* is subsequently obtained from the sample, usually takes one to three days. The time required to ship *E. coli* bacteria from a laboratory to state public health authorities who will perform DNA fingerprinting may take up to a week, depending on the transportation system within a state and the distance between a clinical laboratory and public health department. The time required for state public health officials to perform DNA fingerprinting on an *E. coli* sample and compare it with an outbreak pattern is ideally one day. However, with limited staff and space in public health laboratories during a period when other emergencies may occur, the process can take up to four days.

State health departments typically report laboratory-confirmed cases of foodborne illness to CDC on a regular basis. During serious interstate outbreaks such as the *E. coli* outbreak linked to spinach, state health departments would typically notify CDC of newly confirmed cases on a daily basis, to facilitate a swift nationwide investigation. In general, disease reporting by states to CDC is voluntary, but it may be required as a condition of federal funding for certain state public health systems, such as the PulseNet system described below.

The Systems Used to Monitor Foodborne Illnesses

The tracking and reporting of foodborne illnesses are conducted in several ways:

- PulseNet is a national network of public health and food laboratories coordinated by the CDC. The network consists of labs in state and local health departments and federal agencies (CDC, FDA, and the U.S. Department of Agriculture, or USDA). PulseNet experts perform standardized DNA fingerprinting of foodborne disease-causing bacteria by *pulsed-field gel electrophoresis* (PFGE). PFGE can be used to distinguish among strains of organisms — for example, *E. coli* O157:H7, *Salmonella*, *Shigella*, *Listeria* and *Campylobacter*.[2]

- The OutbreakNet is a group of state public healthofficers who investigate foodborne disease outbreaks and share information throughout an outbreak.
- CDC's Health Alert Network (HAN) is a national program that provides vital health information and the infrastructure to support dissemination of essential information to public health and medical professionals at the state and local levels.
- The Epidemic Information Exchange (Epi-X) is CDC's secure, Web-based communications network that serves as a communications exchange between CDC, state and local health departments, poison control centers, and other public health professionals.

All of these systems have been used in the investigation of the recent *E. coli* outbreak.

Timeline of Cases, Recalls, and Agency Actions[3]

Federal and State Tracking and Investigation

September 8, 2006
According to FDA and CDC reports, the agencies were first alerted on September 8 to four cases of hemolytic uremic syndrome (HUS) in a call from Wisconsin's state epidemiologist. CDC began an investigation, working collaboratively with state health departments and FDA, to detect infections, identify the cause of the infections, and provide information to the public and health care providers on the treatment and prevention of *E. coli* O157:H7 infections.

September 12, 2006

On September 12, the PulseNet system confirmed that the *E. coli* O157:H7 strains from the patients in Wisconsin all had the same DNA fingerprint pattern, and also identified the same pattern in some *E. coli* patients from other states.

September 13, 2006

By September 13, CDC officials were alerted by epidemiologists in Wisconsin and Oregon that fresh spinach was the suspected source of small clusters of *E. coli* cases. The same day, Wisconsin and Oregon epidemiologists were contacted by New Mexico epidemiologists about a cluster of *E. coli* infections that had also been associated with fresh spinach consumption. At this point, the association of illness with spinach consumption was based only on epidemiologic evidence: the common finding, among victims who were interviewed, of a history of recent spinach consumption.

September 14, 2006

FDA and CDC issued the first of nearly three weeks of daily consumer alerts about an *E. coli* outbreak in several states that was believed to be associated with the consumption of fresh produce. At the time, preliminary epidemiological evidence pointed to bagged fresh spinach as the possible cause of the outbreak. FDA advised consumers to avoid consuming bagged spinach. (It is notable that this product-wide advisory was made based solely on epidemiologic evidence, since at this point, the outbreak organism had not yet been identified in any spinach products.) The agencies advised individuals who believed that they had experienced symptoms of illness after consuming bagged spinach to contact their physicians, and physicians were urged to report suspected cases of *E. coli* infection to local and state public healthofficials as soon as possible.

The federal agencies reported that they were working with state and local agencies to determine the cause and scope of the outbreak. Eight states had reported illnesses: Connecticut, Idaho, Indiana, Michigan, Oregon, New Mexico, Utah, and Wisconsin. A total of 50 infected individuals had been identified — among them were eight cases of HUS, one death, and multiple hospitalizations. The date range of infection was estimated to be from August 25 to September 3, 2006.

September 15, 2006

On September 15, FDA and CDC issued announcements that the outbreak of *E. coli* in multiple states had been associated with the consumption of fresh spinach and fresh spinach-containing products. The statements indicated that Natural Selection Foods LLC of San Juan Bautista, California, had launched a voluntary recall of products that contained spinach marked with "best if used by" dates of August 17 through October 1, 2006. (FDA does not have authority to mandate recalls of most of the foods it regulates, including fresh produce.) FDA reported that it was investigating whether eight other companies and their brands were involved. The products under investigation, and subject to an expanded consumer advisory, included spinach and any salad blend containing spinach intended for retail or food service (restaurant and institutional) use. CDC also noted that 94 cases of illness had been reported, and that 29 people (31%) had been hospitalized, 14 (15%) had developed HUS, and one had died.

By this point, California, Kentucky, Maine, Minnesota, Nevada, New York, Ohio, Pennsylvania, Tennessee, Virginia, Washington, and Wyoming had also reported human infections to CDC, bringing the total number of affected states to 20. Spinach from presumptively affected lots was also reported to have been distributed in Canada and Mexico. The agencies also indicated that they, or state officials, were testing available packages of spinach consumed by victims of *E. coli* infection.

September 16, 2006

On September 16, CDC reported that 102 cases of illness due to *E. coli* infection had been confirmed, and that 52 people (51%) had been hospitalized, 16 (16%) had developed HUS, and one had died. Tennessee was removed from the list of states that had confirmed cases because a case originally attributed to the state had actually occurred in Kentucky. FDA advised consumers to avoid fresh bagged spinach, and issued company recall information.

FDA also announced that it was expanding its lettuce safety initiative to cover spinach. In response to repeated *E. coli* outbreaks associated with fresh lettuce, the agency had advised growers in November 2005 of its concerns about the safety of fresh greens, and the need for continued efforts to assure good agricultural and processing practices within the industry.[4] The California Department of Health Services had expressed similar concerns in a letter to California growers in January 2006.[5]

September 17, 2006

On September 17, CDC reported that 109 cases of *E. coli* infection had been confirmed, and that 55 people (50%) had been hospitalized, 16 (15%) had developed HUS, and one had died. FDA announced that a second voluntary recall was under way by the company River Ranch of Salinas, California, which was voluntarily recalling packages of spring mix obtained in bulk from Natural Selection Foods. The FDA's report listed all River Ranch and Natural Selection brands.

September 18, 2006

On September 18, CDC reported that 114 cases of *E. coli* had been confirmed, and that 60 people (53%) had been hospitalized, 18 (16%) had developed HUS, and one had died. CDC added Illinois and Nebraska to the list of states with confirmed cases, bringing the total to 21. The rest of the information reported by CDC and FDA, which was repeated in subsequent notices, was the same as on previous days: consumer advice, symptoms of illness, the two recalls, the lettuce safety initiative and the ongoing investigation.

September 19, 2006

On September 19, CDC reported that the number of *E. coli* cases reported had risen to 131, and that 66 people (50%) had been hospitalized, 20 (15%) had developed HUS, and one had died. FDA stated that products containing tainted spinach had been distributed to Taiwan, as well as to Canada and Mexico (as noted above), but that no illnesses had been reported by those countries.

September 20, 2006

On September 20, CDC reported that the number of reported cases had increased to 146, and that 76 people (52%) had been hospitalized, 23 (16%) had developed HUS, and one had died. Arizona and Colorado had been added to the list of states with confirmed cases, bringing the total to 23. FDA expanded its consumer alert to include fresh spinach in bagged products, spinach in a clamshell, and spinach from farmers' markets. The agency also indicated that it had found no evidence that spinach that was frozen, canned, or an ingredient in pre-made meals manufactured by food companies was tainted. FDA reported a third recall that had been announced by RLB Food Distributors, L.P., of West Caldwell, New Jersey, for certain listed salad products that may have contained spinach with an "enjoy thru" date of September 20, 2006.

The agencies' alerts also noted that the New Mexico Department of Health had announced that through DNA fingerprinting, it had matched a strain of *E. coli* from a victim's package of spinach with the outbreak strain taken from infected patients. This marked the first laboratory confirmation of the link between spinach consumption and *E. coli* infections.

September 21, 2006

On September 21, CDC announced that 157 cases of *E. coli* illness had been reported, and that 83 people (52%) had been hospitalized, 27 (17%) had developed HUS, and one had died. FDA reported that it was working closely with the state of California, since it had been determined that the contaminated spinach had come from fields in the California counties of Monterey, San Benito, and Santa Clara. FDA alerts reassured consumers that processed spinach (frozen and canned) and other produce from those counties were not implicated in the outbreak. The same day, CDC held a Clinician's Outreach and Communication Activity (COCA) conference call with 800 people, who heard experts provide an overview of the current outbreak and FDA's investigation, the nature of *E. coli* as a pathogen, and treatment options for patients exhibiting symptoms of the infection.

September 22, 2006

On September 22, CDC indicated that 166 cases of illness had been reported, and that 88 people (53%) had been hospitalized, 27 (16%) had developed HUS, and one had died. Maryland and Tennessee were added to the list of states with confirmed cases, bringing the total to 25. FDA reported working closely with the state of California in the three counties in which the tainted spinach may have been grown — investigators were attempting to narrow the geographic area suspected of being the source of the outbreak. FDA repeated the consumer notice that processed spinach, spinach grown elsewhere in the United States, and other produce grown in the three implicated counties were safe to eat, and that the food industry was working to get fresh spinach back on the market.

September 23, 2006

On September 23, CDC announced that 171 cases of *E. coli* infection had been reported, and that 92 people (54%) had been hospitalized, 27 (16%) had developed HUS, and one had died. In addition, FDA reported two more voluntary recalls for products containing spinach supplied from Natural Selection Foods of California. Triple B Corporation, doing business as S.T. Produce of Seattle, Washington, recalled its fresh spinach products with "use by" dates of August 22 through September 20, 2006, that had been distributed to retail stores in Idaho, Montana, Oregon, and Washington, and sold in hard plastic clamshell containers. Pacific Coast Fruits Company of Portland, Oregon, recalled products that might contain spinach with "use by" dates of September 20, 2006, or earlier, and on pizza products with dates of September 23, 2006, or earlier. The company reportedly had stopped making all products with spinach supplied from California on September 14, 2006. Its products were shipped to Alaska, Idaho, Oregon, and Washington. For the 25 states with confirmed cases, the number of cases was reported for each state. Hong Kong was added to the list of places outside the U.S. that had received the affected products.

September 24, 2006

On September 24, CDC stated that 173 cases had been reported, and that 92 people (53%) had been hospitalized, 28 (16%) had developed HUS, and one had died. The agencies indicated that the Utah Department of Health and the Salt Lake Valley Health Department had confirmed that *E. coli* O157:H7, the same strain as the one associated with the outbreak, had been found in a bag of Dole baby spinach purchased in Utah with a "use by" date of August 30, 2006. The tests were conducted by the Utah Public Health Laboratory.

September 25, 2006

On September 25, CDC stated that 175 cases had been reported, and that 93 people (53%) had been hospitalized, 28 (16%) had developed HUS, and one had died. FDA reported that tainted products had been distributed to Iceland.

September 26, 2006

On September 26, CDC reported that the number of cases had increased to 183, and that 95 people (52%) had been hospitalized, 29 (16%) had developed HUS, and one had died. West Virginia was added to the list of affected states, bringing the total to 26. CDC and FDA also announced that Canada had reported one confirmed case of *E. coli* O157:H7 that matched the outbreak strain. In addition, they noted that Pennsylvania Department of Health had reported that the outbreak strain of *E. coli* O157:H7 had been isolated from a bag of baby spinach.

September 28, 2006

On September 28, CDC reported that 187 cases infected with the outbreak strain of *E. coli* had been reported, and that 97 people (52%) had been hospitalized, 29 (16%) had developed HUS, and one had died.

September 29, 2006

On September 29, FDA announced that it had determined that spinach implicated in the *E. coli* outbreak had been traced to Natural Selection Foods LLC of San Juan Bautista, California. The determination was based on epidemiologic and laboratory evidence obtained from multiple states (Colorado, Ohio, Wisconsin, Nevada, Pennsylvania, Utah, New Mexico, and Illinois) and analyzed by CDC, and on product distribution information. One company had recalled its product on September 15 and four others had instituted secondary recalls, because they received the recalled product from Natural Selection Foods. The statement indicated that FDA, the state of California, CDC, and the US. Department of Agriculture (USDA) were continuing to investigate the cause of the outbreak through ongoing inspections and sample collections at facilities, in the environment (including irrigation water sources), and through studies of local animal management and water use.

The FDA update indicated that the Grower Shipper Association of Central California, the Produce Marketing Association, the United Fresh Produce Association, and the Western Growers Association had agreed to develop a voluntary plan to improve the safety of fresh produce. FDA and the state of California, however, have not ruled out the possibility of instituting regulatory requirements in the future. In addition, FDA intends to convene a public meeting later in the year to address the larger issue of food-borne illnesses linked to leafy greens once the current investigation is complete.

October 3, 2006

On October 3, CDC reported 192 cases of illness, and that 98 people (51%) had been hospitalized, 30 (16%) had developed HUS, and one died.

October 5, 2006

On October 5, FDA announced that the U.S. Attorney for the Northern District of California had issued a statement on the execution of two search warrants — for Growers Express in Salinas and Natural Selection Foods in San Bautista, California — in connection with the outbreak of *E. coli* O157:H7 that FDA had traced to spinach grown in the Salinas area. The U.S. Attorney stated that there was no indication at that time that leaf spinach had been deliberately or intentionally contaminated. FDA stated that it was working with the U.S. Attorney's office and the Federal Bureau of Investigation (FBI) to determine the facts behind the outbreak, particularly allegations that certain spinach growers and distributors may have failed to take all necessary precautions to ensure that their spinach was safe before it was placed in interstate commerce. The number of reported cases of illness had not changed.

October 6, 2006

On October 6, CDC announced that the number of reported cases had increased to 199 (see figure 1, below) — 102 people (51%) had been hospitalized, and 31 (16%) had developed HUS. On this date, CDC also announced that a total of three people had died in the outbreak — the single case announced earlier, an elderly woman in Wisconsin; and two more victims with E. coli infections that matched the outbreak strain on DNA fingerprinting, a child in Idaho and an elderly woman in Nebraska. CDC also reported a fourth suspicious death in an elderly woman in Maryland, but samples to confirm infection by DNA fingerprinting were not available. The two confirmed deaths announced on this date had occurred in September, but required additional time to link to the outbreak by DNA fingerprinting. CDC reported additional findings as follows:

- Of the individuals affected by the outbreak, 141 (71%) were female and 22 (11%) were children under the age of five.
- The proportions of individuals in each age group who developed HUS included 29% of children under age 18, 8% of those aged 18 to 59, and 14 % of those who were 60 years or older.
- The cases were spread across 26 states: Arizona (8), California (2), Colorado (1), Connecticut (3), Idaho (7), Illinois (2), Indiana (10), Kentucky (8), Maine (3), Maryland (3), Michigan (4), Minnesota (2), Nebraska (11), Nevada (2), New Mexico (5), New York (11), Ohio (25), Oregon (6), Pennsylvania (10), Tennessee (1), Utah (19), Virginia (2), Washington (3), West Virginia (1), Wisconsin (49), and Wyoming (1). (See figure 2, below).

In addition, FDA had determined, based on recall audits, that on September 15, Kenter Canyon Farms, Inc., of Sun Valley, California, had instituted a voluntary recall of repackaged spinach as part of the nationwide recall of Natural Selection Foods. The recalled product was only distributed in California, and carried an expiration date of September 20, 2006.

October 12, 2006

On October 12, FDA and the state of California announced test results from the field investigation of the outbreak of *E. coli* O157:H7 in spinach. Samples of cattle feces taken from one of the four implicated ranches tested positive based on matching DNA fingerprints for the same strain that sickened 199 individuals. The announcement stated that while this finding was significant, it was just one aspect of the trace-back investigation that was ongoing for FDA, the state of California, CDC, and USDA. As of November 8, 2006, this alert was the agencies' most recent. (Readers should note that later news reports[6] have indicated that there were a total of 204 confirmed cases, but this number had not been verified by any available agency documents as of November 8, 2006.)

Developments Following the Agency Alerts on the Outbreak

On October 22, 2006, a statement issued by the United Fresh Produce Association indicated that it understood that FDA had eliminated all concerns about spinach grown anywhere outside of the three counties in California.[7] The group indicated its commitment to determining the specific source of the contamination and working to prevent future outbreaks, including the use of the best agricultural practices in the field and the strongest possible Hazard Analysis and Critical Control Points (HACCP) programs in processing facilities.

The Center for Science in the Public Interest (CSPI) petitioned the state of California to adopt stricter food safety procedures because the state has been at the center of the *E. coli* outbreak, and has experienced other problems with contamination of leafy greens.[8] The petition calls for the California Department of Health Services to establish mandatory regulations relating to manure and water safety on farms, similar to those required of the meat and poultry industries. CSPI suggested that the use of manure as fertilizer should be prohibited during growing season, and that only drinkable water should be used in produce processing facilities.

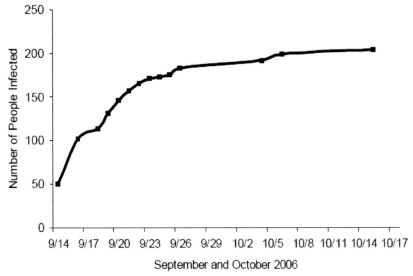

Source: CDC and FDA data; compiled by CRS.

Figure 1. Cumulative Number of *E. coli* Cases Reported by CDC.

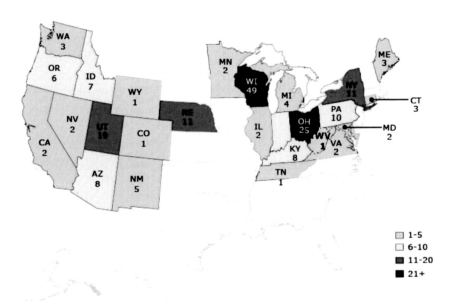

Source: Information provided by CDC. Map adapted by CRS.

Figure 2. Number of Confirmed *E. coli* Cases by State as of October 6, 2006.

On October 29, 2006, a news article reported that the investigation of the *E. coli*spinach outbreak had been thorough, although there were no final answers yet.[9] The article indicated that the codes printed on the bags of spinach had reportedly led detectives to discover when it had been bagged — on August 15 — and other specific details, including worker shift and packing line. Exhaustive testing of the plants' equipment and water supply over several weeks turned up none of the implicated bacteria, according to government officials and company representatives. Company records led investigators to the fields of nine farms in the three counties where the spinach packed on August 15 had been grown. Coding on additional bags of contaminated spinach allowed investigators to narrow the search to four fields. FDA reported that the strain of *E. coli* had been found in manure on a cattle ranch in the SalinasValley, within a mile of spinach fields. Investigators combed the fields for more samples, including wildlife and cattle feces, stream water, and spinach leaves. Six samples taken from the ranch tested positive for the *E. coli* strain that was being sought, including one found in the gut of a feral pig killed on the property. There were also signs that feral pigs had broken through a wire mesh fence to reach the spinach, indicating that the field was a likely source of the outbreak and that the wild pigs were the probable carriers of the bacteria. However, other fields have not been ruled out as the source. Nevertheless, this investigation has provided the most specific information to date for how a microscopic organism commonly found in an animal's feces can cause illness and death in consumers thousands of miles away from the primary source of the contamination.

On October 30, 2006, the Western Growers Association proposed that farmers who grow leafy greens be subject to new food safety standards.[10] While a detailed plan has yet to be released, the statement indicated that soil, irrigation water, and farm equipment should be tested for bacteria, workers should be trained in food safety practices, and processing plants should be checked regularly. Violators could be fined or banned from shipping. The association indicated that the produce industry is subject to little oversight by state and federal regulators, an arrangement that is believed to have led to the *E. coli* outbreak. Losses to the spinach industry alone from the recent outbreak have been estimated to exceed $100 million.[11]

The association proposes to fund the food safety measures through the novel use of a marketing order. Marketing orders were authorized by state and federal legislation in 1937 as a way to compel producers of a particular crop to follow a common set of rules and pay fees used to fund programs. While marketing orders have never been used to enforce food safety, California

Department of Food and Agriculture officials have said that such procedures appear to be within the scope of the law. No information is available on the cost of implementing such a program. Although farmers have to approve marketing orders, they do seem to support the call for increased regulation. The September 2006 outbreak represented the ninth outbreak in California in a decade, and the 20th report of an *E. coli* outbreak in lettuce or leafy greens nationwide since 1995. FDA has reportedly pressed the lettuce and spinach growing industry for more than two years to follow voluntary federal guidelines to prevent outbreaks of foodborne diseases.

On November 2, 2006, a rancher in San Benito County, California, revealed that his operation was one of four farms under investigation by government agencies in connection with the September 2006 *E. coli* outbreak.[12] The rancher indicated that his operation did not grow or process the spinach in question, but that he rented fields to two tenants, one of whom was still under investigation as of November 8. Also on November 2, the Canadian government lifted its ban on U.S. spinach that is grown anywhere outside of San Benito and Monterey counties. Mexico had reportedly lifted its ban on California-grown lettuce in October.

On November 2, 2006, several major supermarkets told growers that they had six weeks to establish new safety rules to prevent *E. coli* outbreaks.[13] The consortium of stores (Vons, Ralph's, and Albertsons grocery chains, and the Costco Wholesale Corporation) wanted growers to work with federal regulators, academia, and industry research scientists to standardize food safety requirements. The group also called for a process for updating food safety rules in response to the emergence of research findings on how diseases are spread from the farm to the dinner table. If growers failed to achieve more stringent and enforceable farming practices, the consortium indicated that it was prepared to set up its own certification system.

Related Congressional Activities

On October 24, 2006, the House Committee on Energy and Commerce asked FDA to explain its role in detecting contaminated food, particularly the *E. coli* strain that tainted spinach in September 2006.[14] The request asked for detailed information about the agency's food contamination preparedness and deterrence assessment, conducted in 2004, and how the assessment was being used in emergencies like the 2006 *E. coli* outbreak. The committee's letter asked the agency for the types of food commodities selected for vulnerability assessments under its 2004 assessment, known as the FDA Security Surveillance Assignment (FSSA), and how the data were collected and analyzed. (FSSA was conducted to determine the safety of food at special security events, such as the G-8 Summit and the national political conventions.)

The recent *E. coli* outbreak led opponents of the National Uniformity for Food Act (S. 3128, H.R. 4167), which is scheduled to come before the Senate in the closing days of the 109th Congress, to call for a rejection of the bill. The Association of Food and Drug Officials (AFDO) has indicated that states' ability to react to future bacterial outbreaks would be compromised. While FDA does not have authority to mandate recalls for most of the foods it regulates, the states generally do have this authority. Proponents of the bill argue that the legislation would not affect state adulteration or inspection authorities. Supporters believe that state food regulators are simply wrong to say that the legislation standardizing food warning labels would have hindered states' ability to recall spinach. See CRS Report RL33559, *Food Safety: National Uniformity for Food Act*, by Donna V. Porter, for further information.

The House and Senate Agriculture Committees may address the recent outbreak of foodborne illness that occurred as a result of spinach contaminated by *E. coli,* possibly from animal manure, when they take up reauthorization of the farm bill in the 110th Congress. Some members have been longtime critics of the division of food safety responsibilities between USDA, which regulates meat, poultry, and processed egg products, and FDA, which regulates all other food products. A proposal for a single food safety agency with increased powers may become part of the debate.

While not mentioned in FDA's reports of its investigation, it is likely that the investigation was streamlined as a result of certain new authorities granted to FDA in comprehensive bioterrorism and public healthpreparedness legislation in the 107th Congress. P.L. 107-188, the Public Health Security and Bioterrorism Preparedness and Response Act of 2002, gave FDA the authority to require that food processing facilities register with the agency, which had not been previously required. In addition, processors were required to maintain records that FDA could use to facilitate product trace-backs during outbreak investigations, including in their records information about the source of ingredients coming into their facilities ("one step back") and the customers to whom they shipped products ("one step forward").

Final Observations

The federal and state systems for tracking and investigating the bacterial outbreak seem to have worked well once the clusters of *E. coli* infections were recognized in several states. Investigators were able to trace back to the likely location and source of the problem through a mix of epidemiologic and laboratory investigation, and multi-agency coordination. The FDA and CDC provided alerts to the public and to health officials, and continued to do so through daily updates. In addition, CDC held a conference call for 800 health care professionals on the investigation of the outbreak, *E. coli* testing, and treatment of patients.

A weak point in the system seems to be how best to intercept *E. coli* contamination before it enters the food chain. While procedures are in place to enhance the safety of meat products, the voluntary federal guidelines for leafy greens seem to be ineffective or not fully implemented by growers and processors. Plans to develop a more effective system announced by the produce industry may address this weakness in the food chain. However, mandatory requirements may need to be implemented by regulators to assure the public that leafy greens are safe for consumption. While funding through market orders has been proposed by one group, the question of whether this source of funding or another source is used remains to be resolved. Oversight of the produce safety system will likely be needed.

In the final analysis, the specific cause of the California spinach *E. coli* outbreak may never be known. Investigators were able to develop a fairly good idea of how the contamination and outbreak occurred, thanks to identifying information on bagged spinach, and DNA fingerprinting technology. While livestock and feral pigs were shown to be carriers of the implicated *E. coli* strain, the precise pathway by which the spinach became contaminated is as yet unclear. Best agricultural practices and HACCP in processing operations are likely to help in preventing such outbreaks in the future.

References

[1]   CDC. (2006). "Timeline for Reporting of Cases with the Outbreak Strain of E. coli O157," Sept. 19, at
      [http://www.cdc.gov/foodborne/ecolispinach/reportingtimeline.htm].

[2]   CDC, PulseNet home page, at [http://www.cdc.gov/pulsenet/index.htm].

[3]   The data in this section were taken from the daily alerts issued by FDA
        and CDC, available at the following sites:
        [http://www.fda.gov/oc/opacom/ hottopics/spinach.html] and
        [http://www.cdc.gov/foodborne/ecolispinach/].

[4]   FDA. (2006). "Nationwide *E. coli* O157:H7 Outbreak: Questions and
        Answers," Sept. 16, at [http://www.cfsan.fda.gov/~dms/spinacqa.html].

[5]   California Department of Health Services, "CDHS *E. coli* Information
        Website," at [http://www.dhs.ca.gov/opa/ecoli/].

[6]   "Turning over a new leaf: Produce group wants farmers to foot the bill
        for inspections." *The Sacramento Bee*, October 31, 2006.

[7]   "Escherichia coli O157:H7 outbreak investigation narrows," Medical
        Letter on the CDC and FDA via NewsRx.com and NewRx.net, Oct. 22,
        2006.

[8]   Center for Science in the Public Interest, "California urged to monitor
        farms for food safety," Oct. 25, 2006, at [http://www.cspinet.org/new/
        200610251.html].

[9]   "Spinach probe most thorough ever, but no clear answers yet," *The
        Associated Press*, State and Local Wire, Oct. 29, 2006.

[10]   See: Western Growers Association, "Western Growers Board Takes
        Action To Require Mandatory Food Safety Practices," press release,
        Oct. 30, 2006, at [http://www.wga.com/public/active
        /siteBuilder/templateNews ReleasePopup.php?id=70]; and "Turning
        over a new leaf: Produce group wants farmers to foot the bill for
        inspections." *The Sacramento Bee*, Oct. 31, 2006.

[11]   Ibid.

[12]   One of four farms under investigation named. (2006). *The Californian*
        (Salinas, California), Nov. 2.

[13]   "Grocers enter produce-safety debate: Big supermarket chains tell
        growers they have six weeks to create rules to avoid E.coli outbreaks."
        The Los Angeles Times, November 2, 2006.

[14]   House Committee on Energy and Commerce. (2006). "Oversight letter
        to the FDA concerning the safety of the U.S. food supply and the
        adequacy of the FDA's food safety and food security efforts,"letter to
        Dr. Andrew C von Eschenbach, FDA Commissioner, Oct. 24, at
        [http://energycommerce. house.gov/108/letters/letters.htm].

In: Foodborne Illness, E. coli and Salmonella   ISBN: 978-1-62100-052-5
Editors: M. Laskaris and F. Korol   © 2011 Nova Science Publishers, Inc.

Chapter 3

Frequently Asked Questions about Escherichia coli O157:H7 and other Shiga Toxin-Producing *Escherichia coli* (STEC)

Marion Laskaris and Fred Korol

What is *Escherichia coli*?

Escherichia coli (abbreviated as *E. coli*) are a large and diverse group of bacteria. Although most strains of *E. coli* are harmless, others can make you sick. Some kinds of *E. coli* can cause diarrhea, while others cause urinary tract infections, respiratory illness and pneumonia, and other illnesses. Still other kinds of *E. coli* are used as markers for water contamination—so you might hear about *E. coli* being found in drinking water, which are not themselves harmful, but indicate the water is contaminated. It does get a bit confusing—even to microbiologists.

What are Shiga Toxin-producing *E. coli*?

Some kinds of *E. coli* cause disease by making a toxin called Shiga toxin. The bacteria that make these toxins are called "Shiga toxin-producing" *E. coli*, or STEC for short. You might hear them called verocytotoxic *E. coli* (VTEC) or enterohemorrhagic *E. coli* (EHEC); these all refer generally to the same group of bacteria. The most commonly identified STEC in North America is *E. coli* O157:H7 (often shortened to *E. coli* O157 or even just "O157"). When you hear news reports about outbreaks of "*E. coli*" infections, they are usually talking about *E. coli* O157.

In addition to *E. coli* O157, many other kinds (called serogroups) of STEC cause disease. These other kinds are sometimes called "non-O157 STEC." *E. coli* serogroups O26, O111, and O103 are the non-O157 serogroups that most often cause illness in people in the United States.

Are there Important Differences between *E. coli* O157 and Other STEC?

Most of what we know about STEC comes from outbreak investigations and studies of *E. coli* O157 infection, which was first identified as a pathogen in 1982. The non-O157 STEC are not nearly as well understood, partly because outbreaks due to them are rarely identified. As a whole, the non-O157 serogroup is less likely to cause severe illness than *E. coli* O157; however, some non-O157 STEC serogroups can cause the most severe manifestations of STEC illness.

Who Gets STEC Infections?

People of any age can become infected. Very young children and the elderly are more likely to develop severe illness and hemolytic uremic syndrome (HUS) than others, but even healthy older children and young adults can become seriously ill.

What Are the Symptoms of STEC Infections?

The symptoms of STEC infections vary for each person but often include severe stomach cramps, diarrhea (often bloody), and vomiting. If there is fever, it usually is not very high (less than 101°F/less than 38.5°C). Most people get better within 5–7 days. Some infections are very mild, but others are severe or even life-threatening.

What Are the Complications of STEC Infections?

Around 5–10% of those who are diagnosed with STEC infection develop a potentially life-threatening complication known as hemolytic uremic syndrome (HUS). Clues that a person is developing HUS include decreased frequency of urination, feeling very tired, and losing pink color in cheeks and inside the lower eyelids. Persons with HUS should be hospitalized because their kidneys may stop working and they may develop other serious problems. Most persons with HUS recover within a few weeks, but some suffer permanent damage or die.

How Soon Do Symptoms Appear after Exposure?

The time between ingesting the STEC bacteria and feeling sick is called the "incubation period." The incubation period is usually 3-4 days after the exposure, but may be as short as 1 day or as long as 10 days. The symptoms often begin slowly with mild belly pain or non-bloody diarrhea that worsens over several days. HUS, if it occurs, develops an average 7 days after the first symptoms, when the diarrhea is improving.

Where Do STEC Come from?

STEC live in the guts of ruminant animals, including cattle, goats, sheep, deer, and elk. The major source for human illnesses is cattle. STEC that cause human illness generally do not make animals sick. Other kinds of animals, including pigs and birds, sometimes pick up STEC from the environment and may spread it.

How Are these Infections Spread?

Infections start when you swallow STEC—in other words, when you get tiny (usually invisible) amounts of human or animal feces in your mouth. Unfortunately, this happens more often than we would like to think about. Exposures that result in illness include consumption of contaminated food, consumption of unpasteurized (raw) milk, consumption of water that has not been disinfected, contact with cattle, or contact with the feces of infected people. Some foods are considered to carry such a high risk of infection with *E. coli* O157 or another germ that health officials recommend that people avoid them completely. These foods include unpasteurized (raw) milk, unpasteurized apple cider, and soft cheeses made from raw milk. Sometimes the contact is pretty obvious (working with cows at a dairy or changing diapers, for example), but sometimes it is not (like eating an undercooked hamburger or a contaminated piece of lettuce). People have gotten infected by swallowing lake water while swimming, touching the environment in petting zoos and other animal exhibits, and by eating food prepared by people who did not wash their hands well after using the toilet. Almost everyone has some risk of infection.

Where Did *My* Infection Come from?

Because there are so many possible sources, for most people we can only guess. If your infection happens to be part of the about 20% of cases that are part of a recognized outbreak, the health department might identify the source.

How Common Are STEC Infections?

An estimated 265,000 STEC infections occur each year in the United States. STEC O157 causes about 36% of these infections, and non-O157 STEC cause the rest. Public health experts rely on estimates rather than actual numbers of infections because not all STEC infections are diagnosed, for several reasons. Many infected people do not seek medical care; many of those who do seek care do not provide a stool specimen for testing, and many labs do not test for non-O157 STEC. However, this situation is changing as more labs have begun using newer, simpler tests that can help detect non-O157 STEC.

How Are STEC Infections Diagnosed?

STEC infections are usually diagnosed through laboratory testing of stool specimens (feces). Identifying the specific strain of STEC is essential for public health purposes, such as finding outbreaks. Many labs can determine if STEC are present, and most can identify *E. coli* O157. Labs that test for the presence of Shiga toxins in stool can detect non-O157 STEC infections. However, for the O group (serogroup) and other characteristics of non-O157 STEC to be identified, Shiga toxin-positive specimens must be sent to a state public health laboratory.

How Long Can an Infected Person Carry STEC?

STEC typically disappear from the feces by the time the illiness is resolved, but may be shed for several weeks, even after symptoms go away. Young children tend to carry STEC longer than adults. A few people keep shedding these bacteria for several months. Good hand-washing is always a smart idea to protect yourself, your family, and other persons.

What Is the Best Treatment for STEC Infection?

Non-specific supportive therapy, including hydration, is important. Antibiotics should not be used to treat this infection. There is no evidence that treatment with antibiotics is helpful, and taking antibiotics may increase the risk of HUS. Antidiarrheal agents like Imodium® may also increase that risk.

Should an Infected Person Be Excluded from School or Work?

School and work exclusion policies differ by local jurisdiction. Check with your local or state health department to learn more about the laws where you live. In any case, good hand-washing after changing diapers, after using the toilet, and before preparing food is essential to prevent the spread of these and many other infections.

How Can STEC Infections Be Prevented?

1. WASH YOUR HANDS thoroughly after using the bathroom or changing diapers and before preparing or eating food. WASH YOUR HANDS after contact with animals or their environments (at farms, petting zoos, fairs, even your own backyard).
2. COOK meats thoroughly. Ground beef and meat that has been needle-tenderized should be cooked to a temperature of at least 160°F/70°C. It's best to use a thermometer, as color is not a very reliable indicator of "doneness."
3. AVOID raw milk, unpasteurized dairy products, and unpasteurized juices (like fresh apple cider).
4. AVOID swallowing water when swimming or playing in lakes, ponds, streams, swimming pools, and backyard "kiddie" pools.
5. PREVENT cross contamination in food preparation areas by thoroughly washing hands, counters, cutting boards, and utensils after they touch raw meat.

In: Foodborne Illness, E. coli and Salmonella   ISBN: 978-1-62100-052-5
Editors: M. Laskaris and F. Korol   © 2011 Nova Science Publishers, Inc.

Chapter 4

Recommendations for Diagnosis of Shiga Toxin-Producing *Escherichia coli* Infections by Clinical Laboratories

Morbidity and Mortality Weekly Report

Summary

Shiga toxin–producing *Escherichia coli* (STEC) are a leading cause of bacterial enteric infections in the United States. Prompt, accurate diagnosis of STEC infection is important because appropriate treatment early in the course of infection might decrease the risk for serious complications such as renal damage and improve overall patient outcome. In addition, prompt laboratory identification of STEC strains is essential for detecting new and emerging serotypes, for effective and timely outbreak responses and control measures, and for monitoring trends in disease epidemiology. Guidelines for laboratory identification of STEC infections by clinical laboratories were published in 2006 (1). This report provides comprehensive and detailed recommendations for STEC testing by clinical laboratories, including the recommendation that all stools submitted for routine testing from patients with acute community-acquired diarrhea (regardless of patient age, season of the year, or presence or absence of blood in the stool) be simultaneously cultured for *E. coli* O157:H7 (O157 STEC) and tested with an assay that detects Shiga toxins to detect non-

O157 STEC. The report also includes detailed procedures for specimen selection, handling, and transport; a review of culture and nonculture tests for STEC detection; and clinical considerations and recommendations for management of patients with STEC infection. Improving the diagnostic accuracy of STEC infection by clinical laboratories should ensure prompt diagnosis and treatment of these infections in patients and increase detection of STEC outbreaks in the community.

Introduction

Shiga toxin–producing *E. coli* (STEC) cause approximately 100,000 illnesses, 3,000 hospitalizations, and 90 deaths annually in the United States, according to the last estimate in 1999 [2]. Most reported STEC infections in the United States are caused by *E. coli* O157:H7, with an estimated 73,000 cases occurring each year [2]. Non-O157 STEC bacteria also are important causes of diarrheal illness in the United States; at least 150 STEC serotypes have been associated with outbreaks and sporadic illness [2–4]. In the United States, six non-O157 serogroups (O26, O45, O103, O111, O121, and O145) account for the majority of reported non-O157 STEC infections [5].

The toxins produced by STEC were named based on their similarity in structure and function to Shiga toxins produced by Shigella dystenteriae type 1 [6]. Shiga toxin 1 (Stx1) is neutralized by antibodies against Shiga toxin, whereas Shiga toxin 2 (Stx2) is not neutralized by antibodies against Shiga toxin but is neutralized by homologous antibodies. STEC are also referred to as verocytotoxigenic *E. coli*; STEC that cause human illness are also referred to as enterohemorrhagic *E. coli*. In this report, all *E. coli* that produce a Shiga toxin are referred to as STEC. STEC serotypes are named according to their somatic (O) and flagellar (H) antigens. In this report, all STEC with the O antigen 157 are referred to as O157 STEC, regardless of whether the H7 antigen has been identified or Shiga toxin production has been confirmed. STEC with other O antigens are referred to as non-O157 STEC or by their specific O antigen.

STEC infection causes acute, often bloody, diarrhea. Approximately 8% of persons who receive a diagnosis of O157 STEC infection develop hemolytic uremic syndrome (HUS), a life-threatening condition characterized by thrombocytopenia, hemolytic anemia, and renal failure [7–9]. Thrombotic thrombocytopenic purpura (TTP), a syndrome with signs and symptoms that are similar to those of HUS, is typically diagnosed in adults. When TTP is diagnosed after a diarrheal illness, the condition is usually caused by infection with O157 STEC or another STEC. In this report, regardless of the age of the patient, TTP diagnosed after a diarrheal illness is referred to as HUS [10].

Whether an illness progresses to HUS depends on strain virulence and host factors [11]. Although most persons with diarrhea-associated HUS have an O157 STEC infection, certain non-O157 STEC strains also can lead to HUS [3]. The virulence of non-O157 STEC is partly determined by the toxins they produce; non-O157 STEC strains that produce only Stx2 are more often associated with HUS than strains that produce only Stx1 or that produce both Stx1 and Stx2 [12]. STEC infections and HUS occur in persons of all ages, but the incidence of STEC infection is highest in children aged <5 years, as is the risk for HUS [9]. Although STEC infections are more common during summer months, they can occur throughout the year.

STEC transmission occurs through consumption of a wide variety of contaminated foods, including undercooked ground beef, unpasteurized juice, raw milk, and raw produce (e.g., lettuce, spinach, and alfalfa sprouts); through ingestion of contaminated water; through contact with animals or their environment; and directly from person to person (e.g., in childcare settings). Both O157 STEC and O111 STEC have a low infectious dose (<100 organisms) [13]; the infectious dose of other serogroups is not known.

Prompt and accurate diagnosis of STEC infection is important because appropriate treatment with parenteral volume expansion early in the course of infection might decrease renal damage and improve patient outcome [14]. In addition, because antibiotic therapy in patients with STEC infections might be associated with more severe disease, prompt diagnosis is needed to ensure proper treatment. Furthermore, prompt laboratory identification of STEC strains is essential for implementation of control measures, for effective and timely outbreak responses, to detect new and emerging serotypes, and to monitor trends in disease epidemiology [1,15,16].

Most O157 STEC isolates can be readily identified in the laboratory when grown on sorbitol-containing selective media because O157 STEC cannot ferment sorbitol within 24 hours. However, many clinical laboratories do not routinely culture stool specimens for O157 STEC. In addition, selective and differential media are not available for the culture of non-O157 STEC, and even fewer laboratories culture stool specimens for these bacteria than for O157 STEC.

Recently, the increased use of enzyme immunoassay (EIA) or polymerase chain reaction (PCR) to detect Shiga toxin or the genes that encode the toxins (stx1 and stx2) has facilitated the diagnosis of both O157 and non-O157 STEC infections. Although EIA and other nonculture tests are useful tools for diagnosing STEC infection, they should not replace culture; a pure culture of the pathogen obtained by the clinical laboratory (O157 STEC) or the public health laboratory (non-O157 STEC) is needed for serotyping and molecular characterization (e.g., pulsed-field gel electrophoresis [PFGE] patterns), which are essential for detecting, investigating, and controlling STEC outbreaks.

Simultaneous culture of stool for O157 STEC and EIA testing for Shiga toxin is more effective for identifying STEC infections than the use of either technique alone [17,18]. Because virtually all O157 STEC have the genes for Stx2 (stx2) and intimin (eae), which are found in strains that are associated with severe disease [5,12,19–22], detection of O157 STEC should prompt immediate initiation of steps such as parenteral volume expansion to reduce the risk for renal damage in the patient and the spread of infection to others.

Guidelines for clinical and laboratory identification of STEC infections have been previously published [1]; this report provides the first comprehensive and detailed recommendations for isolation and identification of STEC by clinical laboratories. The recommendations are intended primarily for clinical laboratories but also are an important reference for health-care providers, public health laboratories, public health authorities, and patients and their advocates.

Recommendation for Identification of STEC by Clinical Laboratories

All stools submitted for testing from patients with acute community-acquired diarrhea (i.e., for detection of the enteric pathogens *Salmonella, Shigella,* and *Campylobacter*) should be cultured for O157 STEC on selective and differential agar. These stools should be simultaneously assayed for non-O157 STEC with a test that detects the Shiga toxins or the genes encoding these toxins. All O157 STEC isolates should be forwarded as soon as possible to a state or local public health laboratory for confirmation and additional molecular characterization (i.e., PFGE analysis and virulence gene characterization). Detection of STEC or Shiga toxin should be reported promptly to the treating physician, to the public health laboratory for confirmation, isolation, and subsequent testing of the organism, and to the appropriate public health authorities for case investigation. Specimens or enrichment broths in which Shiga toxin or STEC are detected but from which

O157 STEC are not recovered should be forwarded as soon as possible to a state or local public health laboratory.

Benefits of Recommended Testing Strategy

Identification of Additional STEC Infections and Detection of All STEC Serotypes

Evidence indicates that STEC might be detected as frequently as other bacterial pathogens. In U.S. studies, STEC were detected in 0%–4.1% of stools submitted for testing at clinical laboratories, rates similar to those of *Salmonella species* (1.9%–4.8%), Shigella species (0.2%–3.1%), and Campylobacter species (0.9%–9.3%) [9,17,23–31]. In one study, the proportion of stools with STEC detected varied by study site [9]; O157 STEC were more commonly isolated than some other enteric pathogens in northern states. The laboratory strategy of culturing stool while simultaneously testing for Shiga toxin is more sensitive than other strategies for STEC identification and ensures that all STEC serotypes will be detected [17,18,30,31] (Table 1). In addition, immediate culture ensures that O157 STEC bacteria are detected within 24 hours of the initiation of testing.

Early Diagnosis and Improved Patient outcome

Early diagnosis of STEC infection is important for determining the proper treatment promptly. Initiation of parenteral volume expansion early in the course of O157 STEC infection might decrease renal damage and improve patient outcome (14]. Conversely, certain treatments can worsen patient outcomes; for example, antibiotics might increase the risk for HUS in patients infected with O157 STEC, and antidiarrheal medications might worsen the illness [32]. Early diagnosis of STEC infection also might prevent unnecessary procedures or treatments (e.g., surgery or corticosteroids for patients with severe abdominal pain or bloody diarrhea) [33–35].

Prompt Detection of outbreaks

Prompt laboratory diagnosis of STEC infection facilitates rapid subtyping of STEC isolates by public health laboratories and submission of PFGE patterns to PulseNet, the national molecular subtyping network for foodborne disease surveillance [36]. Rapid laboratory diagnosis and subtyping of STEC isolates leads to prompt detection of outbreaks, timely public health actions, and detection of emerging STEC strains [37,38]. Delayed diagnosis of STEC infections might lead to secondary transmission in homes, child-care settings, nursing homes, and food service establishments [39,40–44] and might delay detection of multistate outbreaks related to widely distributed foods [39,45]. Outbreaks caused by STEC with multiple serogroups (46) or PFGE patterns [47] have been documented.

Criteria for STEC Testing and Specimen Selection

All stool specimens from patients with acute onset of community-acquired diarrhea and from patients with possible HUS should be tested for STEC. Many infections are missed with selective STEC testing strategies (e.g., testing only specimens from children, testing only during summer months, or testing only stools with white blood cells or blood). Some patients with STEC infection do not have visibly bloody stools, whereas some persons infected with other pathogens do have bloody stools [3,9,48,49]. Therefore, the absence of blood in the stool does not rule out the possibility of a STEC-associated diarrheal illness; both O157 and non-O157 strains have been isolated from patients with nonbloody diarrhea [30–32,49–51]. Similarly, white blood cells are often but not always detected in the stools of patients with STEC infection and should not be used as a criterion for STEC testing [9,39]. Selective testing on the basis of patient age or season of the year also might result in undetected infections. Although STEC bacteria are isolated more frequently from children, almost half of all STEC isolates are from persons aged >12 years [5,9,49,52]; testing for STEC only in specimens from children would result in many missed infections. In addition, although STEC infections are more common in summer months, infections and outbreaks occur throughout the year [5,9,32].

Table 1. Comparison of Laboratory Testing Strategies for Shiga Toxin–Producing *Escherichia coli* (STEC)

Testing method*	O157 STEC Confirmed within 24 hrs	O157 STEC Isolate obtained within 24 hrs	Shiga toxin–Negative variants of O157 STEC detected	Sorbitol-Fermenting variants of O157 STEC detected	All STEC serotypes Detected within 24 hrs	Shiga toxin–positive sample available for isolation of STEC within 24 hrs	Comments
Simultaneous culture for O157 STEC and nonculture assay for Shiga toxin	Yes	Yes	Yes	Yes	Yes	Yes	• Recommended practice
Nonculture assay for Shiga toxin followed by culture for O157 STEC if Shiga toxin assay is positive	No	No	No	Yes	Yes	Yes	• Delays detection and isolation of O157 STEC • Delays forwarding of Shiga toxin–positive broths for isolation of non-O157 STEC • Misses O157 STEC that are not actively expressing toxin or have lost Shiga toxin genes
Nonculture assay for Shiga toxin with rapid submission to public health laboratory	No	No	No	Yes	Yes	Yes	• Delays detection and isolation of O157 STEC • Misses O157 STEC that are not expressing toxin or have lost Shiga toxin genes
Culture for O157 STEC	Yes	Yes	Yes	No	No	No	• Misses sorbitol-fermenting variants of O157 STEC • Misses non-O157 STEC

* Performance characteristics reflect use of nonculture assays for Shiga toxin with overnight enrichment broths or growth from the primary isolation plate. Enrichment broths are strongly recommended for the routine diagnostic testing of fecal specimens with nonculture Shiga toxin tests. Because stool specimens can contain inhibitors and might have few target organisms, the sensitivity of nonculture Shiga toxin tests when performed directly on stool specimens is generally insufficient to reliably exclude infection with the target organism (Source: Cornick NA, Jelacic S, Ciol MA, Tarr PI. *Escherichia coli* O157:H7 infections: discordance between filterable fecal Shiga toxin and disease outcome. J Infect Dis 2002;186:57–63.)

Stools should be tested as early as possible in the course of illness; bacteria might be difficult or impossible to detect in the stool after 1 week of illness [53,54], and the Shiga toxin genes might be lost by the bacteria [55]. In certain instances, retrieval of plates from cultures obtained earlier in the illness that were not initially evaluated for STEC might be necessary. Early detection of STEC and proper patient management are especially important among children because they are the age group most likely to have an infection that develops into HUS [32].

STEC testing might not be warranted, or selective STEC testing might be appropriate, for patients who have been hospitalized for ≥3 days; infection in this setting is more likely to be caused by *Clostridium difficile* toxin than another enteric pathogen [39]. However, when a patient is admitted to the hospital with symptoms of a diarrheal illness, a stool culture with STEC testing might be appropriate, regardless of the number of days of hospitalization. In addition, although few hospital-associated outbreaks of STEC have been reported, if a hospitalized patient is involved in a hospital-associated outbreak of diarrhea, STEC testing should be performed if tests are also being conducted for other bacterial enteric pathogens (e.g., Salmonella). Although chronic diarrhea is uncommon in patients with STEC infection, certain STEC strains have been associated with prolonged or intermittent diarrhea; therefore, testing for Shiga toxin should be considered if an alternative diagnosis (e.g., ulcerative colitis) has not been identified [56]. Testing multiple specimens is likely unnecessary unless the original specimen was not transported or tested appropriately or the test results are not consistent with the patient's signs and symptoms. After STEC bacteria are detected in a specimen, additional specimens from the same patient do not need to be tested for diagnostic purposes.

To prevent additional transmission of infection, certain persons (e.g., food-service workers and children who attend child-care facilities or adults who work in these facilities) who receive a diagnosis of STEC infection might be required by state law or a specific facility to prove that they are no longer shedding the bacteria after treatment and before returning to the particular setting. Follow-up specimens are usually tested by state public health laboratories. No data exist regarding the effectiveness of excluding postsymptomatic carriers of non- O157 STEC (i.e., persons who test positive for non-O157 STEC but no longer have symptoms) from work or school settings in preventing secondary spread.

Procedures for Collecting and Handling Specimens for STEC Diagnostic Testing

Acceptable Specimens for Testing

Laboratories should always consult the manufacturer instructions for the assay being performed to determine procedures for specimen collection and handling, including specimen types that may be used with a particular assay or test system. The ideal specimen for testing is diarrheal stool; stool specimens should be collected as soon as possible after diarrhea begins, while the patient is acutely ill, and before any antibiotic treatment is administered. The same specimen that is collected for *Salmonella*, *Shigella*, and *Campylobacter* testing is acceptable for STEC culture and Shiga toxin detection. Collecting and testing specimens as soon as possible after symptom onset is important to ensure maximal sensitivity and specificity for STEC detection with available commercial diagnostic assays. Diagnostic methods such as the Shiga toxin immunoassay that target traits encoded on mobile genetic elements (e.g., phages) are less sensitive if the elements have been lost [53,57].

Shiga toxin testing should be performed on growth from broth culture or primary isolation media because this method is more sensitive and specific than direct testing of stool. In addition, because the amount of free fecal Shiga toxin in stools is often low, EIA testing of broth enrichments from stools or of growth from the primary isolation plate is recommended rather than direct testing of stools [58].

Although rectal swabs are often used to collect stool from children, swabs might not contain enough stool to culture for multiple enteric pathogens and to perform STEC testing. If rectal swabs must be used to collect specimens for STEC testing, broth enrichment is recommended. Laboratories should consult the manufacturer instructions for information on the suitability of toxin testing using stool from rectal swabs.

Commercially available assays have not been validated for specimens collected by endoscopy or colonoscopy. If a laboratory chooses to use an assay for patient testing with a specimen other than that included in the manufacturer's FDA-cleared package insert, under the Clinical Laboratory Improvement Amendments (CLIA) of 1988, that laboratory must first establish the performance specifications for the alternative specimen type [59]. Unless STEC are isolated, results from tests on alternative specimen types should be interpreted with caution.

Specimen Handling

Specimens should be sent to the laboratory as soon as possible for O157 STEC culture and Shiga toxin testing. Ideally, specimens should be processed as soon as they are received by the laboratory. Specimens that are not processed immediately should be refrigerated until tested; if possible, they should not be held for >24 hours unpreserved or for >48 hours in transport medium. All O157 STEC isolates and all specimens or enrichment broths in which Shiga toxin is detected but from which O157 STEC bacteria are not recovered should be forwarded to the public health laboratory as soon as possible in compliance with the receiving laboratory's guidelines.

Transport Media

Specimens should be transported under conditions appropriate for the transport medium used and tests to be performed; appropriate transport conditions can be determined by reviewing the manufacturer instructions. Stool specimens that cannot be immediately transported to the laboratory for testing should be put into a transport medium (e.g., Cary-Blair) that is optimal for the recovery of all bacterial enteric pathogens. Laboratories should consult the manufacturer instructions for the suitability of toxin testing for stool in transport medium. If a laboratory must perform direct Shiga toxin testing of stool, the stool specimen should be refrigerated but should not be placed in transport medium. Direct toxin testing of stool should follow the manufacturer instructions.

Culture for STEC

O 157 STEC

O157 STEC can usually be easily distinguished from most *E. coli* that are members of the normal intestinal flora by their inability to ferment sorbitol within 24 hours on sorbitolcontaining agar isolation media. To isolate O157 STEC, a stool specimen should be plated onto a selective and differential medium such as sorbitol-MacConkey agar (SMAC) [60], cefixime tellurite-sorbitol MacConkey agar (CT-SMAC), or CHROMagar O157. After incubation for 16–24 hours at 37°C (99°F), the plate should be examined for possible O157 colonies, which are colorless on SMAC or CT-SMAC and are mauve or pink on CHROMagar O157. Both CT-SMAC and CHROMagar O157 are more selective than SMAC, which increases the sensitivity of culture for detection of O157 STEC [61,62]. Sorbitol-fermenting STEC O157:H- (i.e., nonmotile [NM]), a pathogen that is uncommon in the United States and primarily reported from Germany, might not grow on CT-SMAC agar because the bacteria are susceptible to tellurite.

To identify O157 STEC, a portion of a well-isolated colony (i.e., a distinct, single colony) should be selected from the culture plate and tested in O157-specific antiserum or O157 latex reagent as recommended by the manufacturer [63]. Colonies that agglutinate with one of the O157-specific reagents and do not agglutinate with normal serum or control latex reagent are presumed to be O157 STEC. At least three colonies should be screened (CDC, unpublished data, 2009). If O157 STEC bacteria are identified in any one of the three colonies, no additional colonies need to be tested.

The colony in which O157 STEC are detected should be streaked onto SMAC or a nonselective agar medium such as tryptic soy agar (TSA), heart infusion agar (HIA), or blood agar and biochemically confirmed to be *E. coli* (e.g., using standard biochemical tests or commercial automated systems) because other bacterial species can cross-react in O157 antiserum [64–66]. Before confirmation is complete at the laboratory (which might take >24 hours), the preliminary finding of O157 STEC should be reported to the treating clinician and should be documented according to laboratory policies for other time-sensitive, clinically important laboratory findings. The preliminary nature of these presumptive results and the need for test confirmation should be indicated in the report. After O157 STEC colonies have been isolated, been found to agglutinate with O157 latex reagent, and been biochemically confirmed as E. coli, a written or electronic report should be provided to the clinician and public health authorities (Table 2).

All O157 STEC isolates should be forwarded to the public health laboratory as soon as possible, regardless of whether H7 testing has been attempted or completed. At the public health laboratory, O157 STEC isolates should be tested by EIA for Shiga toxin production or by PCR for the *stx1* and *stx2* genes. Actively motile O157 STEC strains should be tested for the H7 antigen. All O157 STEC strains should be subtyped by PFGE as soon as possible.

Non-O157 STEC

Identification of non-O157 STEC typically occurs at the public health laboratory and not at clinical laboratories (Table 3). However, this section includes the basic techniques for reference.

To isolate non-O157 STEC, the Shiga toxin–positive broth should be streaked to a relatively less selective agar (e.g., MacConkey agar, SMAC, Statens Serum Institut [SSI] enteric medium, or blood agar). Traditional enteric media such as Hektoen agar, xylose-lysine-desoxycholate agar, and Salmonella-Shigella agar inhibit many *E. coli* and are not recommended [67]. All possible O157 STEC colonies should be tested in O157 latex reagent before isolation of non-O157 STEC is attempted. Well-isolated colonies with *E. coli*-like morphology should be selected on the basis of sorbitol or lactose fermentation characteristics (or other characteristics specific to the medium used); most non-O157 STEC ferment both sorbitol and lactose, although exceptions have been reported (CDC, unpublished data, 2009). Colonies may be tested for Shiga toxin production by EIA or for *stx1* and *stx2* genes by PCR. Non-O157 STEC may be tested using commercial O-specific antisera for the most common STEC-associated O antigens (i.e., O26, O45, O103, O111, O121, and O145) [5]. Non-O157 STEC isolates should be forwarded to a public health laboratory for confirmation of Shiga toxin production, serogroup determination, and PFGE subtyping.

Nonculture Assays for Detection of Shiga Toxins and STEC

Nonculture assays that detect the Shiga toxins produced by STEC (e.g., the Shiga toxin EIA) were first introduced in the United States in 1995. The primary advantage of nonculture assays for Shiga toxin is that they can be used to detect all serotypes of STEC. In addition, nonculture assays might provide results more quickly than culture. The primary disadvantage of nonculture based assays is that the infecting organism is not isolated for subsequent serotyping and a specific diagnosis of O157 STEC. Lack of an isolated organism limits the ability of physicians to predict the potential severity of the infection in the patient (e.g., risk for HUS), the risk for severe illness in patient contacts, and the ability of public health officials to detect and control STEC outbreaks and monitor trends in STEC epidemiology. In addition, although the nonculture assays for Shiga toxin also detect Stx1 produced by *Shigella dysenteriae* type 1, infection with this organism is rare in the United States, with fewer than five cases reported each year [68].

Table 2. Documentation of Shiga Toxin–Producing *Escherichia coli* (STEC) Test Results in Final Laboratory Reports

Test	Result	Examples of documentation in final report
Culture for O157 STEC	Positive	*Escherichia coli* O157:H7 or Shiga toxin–producing *E. coli* O157 isolated
	Negative	*Escherichia coli* O157:H7 or Shiga toxin–producing *E. coli* O157 not isolated
Culture for STEC	Positive	Shiga toxin–producing *Escherichia coli* O___:H_ isolated*
	Negative	Shiga toxin–producing *Escherichia coli* not isolated, suggesting that Shiga toxin–producing *E. coli* is not present
Immunoassay detection of Shiga toxin antigen	Positive	Shiga toxin detected by immunoassay, indicating the likely presence of a Shiga toxin–producing *Escherichia coli* such as *E. coli* O157:H7
	Negative	Shiga toxin not detected by immunoassay, suggesting that a Shiga toxin–producing *Escherichia coli*, such as *E. coli* O157, is not present
Detection of Shiga toxin DNA (i.e., Shiga toxin genes)	Positive for Shiga toxin 1 gene (*stx1*), Shiga toxin 2 gene (*stx2*), or both	Genes for Shiga toxin 1, Shiga toxin 2, or both were detected by polymerase chain reaction, indicating the likely presence of a Shiga toxin–producing *Escherichia coli* such as O157:H7
	Negative for Shiga toxin genes	Shiga toxin genes not detected by polymerase chain reaction, suggesting that a Shiga toxin producing *Escherichia coli*, such as O157, is not present

* Public health laboratories may determine the O antigen or send the specimen to CDC for O antigen and H antigen determination.

Shiga Toxin Immunoassays

The Center for Devices and Radiological Health of the Food and Drug Administration (FDA) has approved several immunoassays for the detection of Shiga toxin in human specimens (Table 4). Because the amount of free fecal Shiga toxin in stools is often low [58], EIA testing of enrichment broth cultures incubated overnight (16–24 hours at 37°C [99°F]), rather than direct testing of stool specimens, is recommended. In addition, the manufacturer information indicates that tests performed on broth cultures have higher sensitivity and specificity than those performed on stool. No studies have determined whether one type of broth is most effective; MacConkey and gram-negative broths are both suitable.

Four FDA-approved immunoassays are available in the United States (Table 4). The Premier EHEC (Meridian Diagnostics, Cincinnati, Ohio) and the ProSpecT Shiga Toxin *E. coli* Microplate Assay (Remel, Lenexa, Kansas) are in a microplate EIA format; the Immunocard STAT! EHEC (Meridian Diagnostics, Cincinnati, Ohio) and the Duopath Verotoxins Gold Labeled Immunosorbent Assay (Merck, Germany) are lateral flow immunoassays. Both the Immunocard STAT! EHEC and the Duopath Verotoxins assays differentiate between Stx1 and Stx2; the Premier EHEC and the ProSpecT assays do not differentiate between Stx1 and Stx2. The time required for these assays, not including the time for overnight enrichment, ranges from 20 minutes to 4 hours, depending on the test format used. Specific instructions and actual requirements for each test can be determined by consulting the manufacturer instructions.

Reported sensitivities and specificities of Shiga toxin immunoassays vary by test format and manufacturer. The standard by which each manufacturer evaluates its tests varies; a direct comparison of performance characteristics of various immunoassays has not been made. The clinical performance characteristics of each test are available in the package insert. Clinical laboratories should evaluate these performance characteristics and verify that they can obtain performance specifications comparable to those of the manufacturer before implementing a particular test system. The College of American Pathologists [69] and the American Proficiency Institute [70] offer proficiency testing for STEC immunoassays.

Table 3. Shiga Toxin–Producing *Escherichia coli* (STEC) Testing Procedures Typically Performed by Clinical and Public Health Laboratories, by Type of Laboratory

Test performed	Testing procedures typically performed[†]	
	Clinical laboratory[†]	Public health laboratory
Culture for O157 STEC	• Specimens plated to selec-tive and differential media • Possible STEC colonies tested for O157 antigen • Biochemical testing per-formed on O157-positive colonies to identify *E. coli* • O157 isolates forwarded to public health laboratory	• O157 antigen confirmed • H7 serology or Shiga toxin antigen or Shiga toxin gene testing performed[§]
Culture for non-O157 STEC	• Not typically performed	• Specimens plated to selective and differential media • Possible STEC colonies tested for Shiga toxin or Shiga toxin genes • Biochemical testing performed of STEC colony to identify *E. coli* • O and H antigen serology performed[¶]
Immunoassay detection of Shiga toxin antigen	• Specimens tested directly or after enrichment by immunoassay according to manufacturer recommendations • Shiga toxin–positive specimens forwarded to public health laboratory	• Specimens retested by immunoassay for evidence of STEC[**] • Shiga toxin–positive specimens cultured for O157 STEC and non-O157 STEC
Detection of Shiga toxin DNA (i.e.,	• Not typically performed	• Specimens tested for Shiga toxin 1 gene (*stx1*) and Shiga toxin 2

Table 3. (Continued)

Test performed	Testing procedures typically performed*	
	Clinical laboratory[†]	**Clinical laboratory**[†]
Shiga toxin genes)		gene (*stx2*) directly or after enrichment[††] • Positive specimens cultured for O157 STEC and non-O157 STEC

* Some testing procedures overlap between clinical and public health laboratories. When risk for STEC transmission to the public is high (e.g., workers in restaurants or child-care facilities), public health laboratories might conduct more of the primary STEC testing.

[†] Simultaneous O157 STEC culture and Shiga toxin testing is recommended. Clinical laboratories should submit all STEC isolates and Shiga toxin–positive broths to a public health laboratory for additional testing.

[§] Before sending the final report, public health laboratories should ensure that the isolated strain has genes for Shiga toxin, produces Shiga toxin, or has the H7 antigen.

[¶] The public health laboratory may determine the O antigen or send the isolate to CDC for O antigen and H antigen determination.

[**] Public health laboratories that detect Shiga toxin by immunoassay are encouraged to use a different manufacturer kit than the one used by the clinical laboratory whose results they are confirming and should request the name of the kit used for each test.

[††] DNA-based Shiga toxin gene detection is not approved by the Food and Drug Administration for diagnosis of human STEC infections by clinical laboratories; however, public health laboratories might use this technique for confirmatory testing after internal validation.

Table 4. Immunoassays Approved by the Food and Drug Administration (FDA) for the Diagnosis of Shiga Toxin–Producing *Escherichia coli* (STEC) Infection

Test	Company	Format	Target	Time	Specimen[*]	Comments	Sensitivity[†] (%)	Specificity[†] (%)
BioStar OIA SHIGATOX[§]	Inverness Medical Professional Diagnostics, Inc. (Boston, Massachusetts)	Optical immunoassay	Shiga toxins; cannot differentiate	15 min	• Direct stool • Enrichment broth • Isolate • Stool in transport medium (Cary-Blair)	Will be withdrawn from the market in 2009	100	98
Duopath Verotoxins Gold Labeled Immunosorbent Assay[¶]	Merck (Germany)	Lateral flow immunoassay	Shiga toxins; can differentiate between 1 and 2	20 min	• Isolate	—	100 (Shiga toxin 1) 99 (Shiga toxin 2)	98 (Shiga toxin 1) 97 (Shiga toxin 2)
Immunocard STAT! EHEC[**]	Meridian Diagnostics, Inc. (Cincinnati, Ohio)	Lateral flow immunoassay	Shiga toxins; can differentiate between 1 and 2	20 min	• Enrichment broth • Isolate	—	92	100
Premier EHEC[††]	Meridian Diagnostics, Inc. (Cincinnati, Ohio)	Microplate enzyme immunoassay (EIA)	Shiga toxins; cannot differentiate between 1 and 2	~3.5 hrs	• Direct stool • Enrichment broth • Isolate	Testing after overnight broth enrichment is recommended; manufacturer instructions for direct testing of stools says relative sensitivity is 79%	100	98

Table 4. (Continued)

Test	Company	Format	Target	Time	Specimen[*]	Comments	Sensitivity[†] (%)	Specificity[†] (%)
ProSpecT Shiga Toxin E. coli Microplate Assay[§§]	Remel (Lenexa, Kansas)	Microplate EIA	Shiga toxins; cannot differentiate between 1 and 2	~3 hrs	• Direct stool • Enrichment broth • Stool in transport medium (Cary-Blair)	Testing after overnight broth enrichment is recommended; manufacturer's insert for direct testing of stools says relative sensitivity is 87%	100	100
VTEC Screen "Seiken"/Den ka Seiken RPLA[¶]	Denka Seiken (Japan)	Reversed passive latex agglutination (RPLA)	Shiga toxins; can differentiate between 1 and 2	4 hrs	• Isolate	Not available in the United States	100	100

[*] Appropriate specimen for testing according to manufacturer recommendations. EIA testing of enrichment broth cultures incubated overnight (16–24 hours at 37°C [99°F]), rather than of stool specimens, is recommended because the amount of free fecal Shiga toxin in stools is often low (Cornick NA, Jelacic S, Ciol MA, Tarr PI. *Escherichia coli* O157:H7 infections: discordance between filterable fecal Shiga toxin and disease outcome. J Infect Dis 2002;186:57–63). In addition, the manufacturer information indicates that tests performed on broth cultures have higher sensitivity and specificity than those performed on stool.

[†] Obtained from the manufacturer's package insert. The standard by which each manufacturer evaluates its tests varies; a direct comparison of performance characteristics has not been made. Clinical laboratories should evaluate these performance characteristics and verify that they can obtain performance specifications comparable to those of the manufacturer before implementing a particular test system. Actual sensitivity and specificity might differ depending on the type of specimen tested.

[§] Test evaluation information available from Teel LD, Daly JA, Jerris RC, et al. Rapid detection of Shiga toxin-producing *Escherichia coli* by optical immunoassay. J Clin Microbiol 2007;45:3377–80.

[¶] Test evaluation information available from Park CH Kim HJ, Hixon DL, Bubert A. Evaluation of the Duopath verotoxin test for detection of Shiga toxins in cultures of human stools. J Clin Microbiol 2003;41:2650–3.

[**] Enterohemorrhagic E. coli. Additional information available at http://www.mdeur.com/products/751630.htm.

†† Test evaluation information available from Kehl K, Havens P, Behnke CE, Acheson DW. Evaluation of the premier EHEC assay for detection of Shiga toxin–producing Escherichia coli. J Clin Microbiol 1997;35:2051–4.

§§ Test evaluation information available from Gavin PJ, Peterson LR, Pasquariello AC, et al. Evaluation of performance and potential clinical impact of ProSpecT Shiga toxin Escherichia coli microplate assay for detection of Shiga toxin–producing E. coli in stool samples. J Clin Microbiol 2004;42:1652–6.

¶ Reversed passive latex agglutination. Test evaluation information available from Carroll KC, Adamson K, Korgenski K, et al. Comparison of a commercial reversed passive latex agglutination assay to an enzyme immunoassay for the detection of Shiga toxin–producing Escherichia coli. Eur J Clin Microbiol Infect Dis 2003;22:689–92; Bettelheim KA. Development of a rapid method for the detection of verocytotoxin-producing Escherichia coli (VTEC). Lett Appl Microbiol 2001;33:31–5; and Beutin L, Zimmermann S, Gleier K. Evaluation of the VTEC-Screen "Seiken" test for detection of different types of Shiga toxin (verotoxin)-producing Escherichia coli (STEC) in human stool samples. Diagn Microbiol Infect Dis 2002;42:1–8.

Laboratories should immediately report Shiga toxin–positive specimens to the treating clinician and appropriate public health and infection control officials. Clinical laboratories should forward Shiga toxin–positive specimens or enrichment broths to a public health laboratory as soon as possible for isolation and additional characterization.

In multiple studies, for reasons that are unknown, EIAs failed to detect a subset of O157 STEC that were readily identified on simultaneously plated SMAC agar, underscoring the importance of primary isolation [17,50,71–73]. EIA tests also might have false-positive STEC results when other pathogens are present [1,74,75].

PCR

PCR assays to detect the *stx1* and *stx2* genes are used by many public health laboratories for diagnosis and confirmation of STEC infection. Depending on the primers used, these assays can distinguish between *stx1* and *stx2* [76–78]. Assays also have been developed that determine the specific O group of an organism, detect virulence factors such as intimin and enterohemolysin, and can differentiate among the subtypes of Shiga toxins [79–81]. Because these tests are not commercially available, they are rarely used for human disease diagnosis in the United States.

Most PCR assays are designed and validated for testing isolated colonies taken from plated media; some assays have been validated for testing on stool specimens subcultured to an enrichment broth and incubated for 18–24 hours. Shiga toxin PCR assays on DNA extracted from whole stool specimens are not recommended because the sensitivity is low [82]. The time required to obtain PCR assay results ranges from 3 hours (if an isolate is tested) to 24–36 hours (if the specimen is first subcultured to an enrichment broth or plate).

DNA-based Shiga toxin gene detection is not approved by FDA for diagnosis of human STEC infections by clinical laboratories; however, public health laboratories might use this technique for confirmatory testing after internal validation. One commercial PCR kit is available to test for STEC virulence genes (DEC Primer Mix, Mira Vista Diagnostics, Indianapolis, Indiana); however, this test is labeled for research use only, can only be used on isolates, and is not approved by FDA for diagnosis of human STEC infections. Clinical laboratories that are considering adding a DNA-based assay to their testing options need to establish performance specifications for the assay as required by CLIA [59], and reports from such testing should include a disclaimer to inform clinicians that the test is not approved by FDA [83]. No commercially available proficiency testing programs are available in the United States for PCR assays that target the Shiga toxin genes; however, internal proficiency testing events and exchanges with other laboratories may be used to fulfill CLIA requirements [84].

O157 Immunoassays

One commercial immunoassay is available to test for the O157 and H7 antigens in human stools and stool cultures (ImmunoCard STAT! *E. coli* O157:H7; Meridian Bioscience, Cincinnati, Ohio). This rapid assay may be performed either directly on stools or on an enrichment broth culture incubated overnight (16–24 hours at 37°C [99°F]). When performed directly on stool specimens, compared with culture for O157 STEC, the assay has an overall sensitivity of 81% and specificity of 97% [85,86]. This test is not recommended as a first-line or primary test for diagnosis, in part because 1) the assay does not detect non-O157 STEC serogroups, 2) not all *E. coli* O157 produce Shiga toxin, and 3) no isolates will be available for testing at the public health laboratory. Laboratories that use this test should ensure that specimens in which O157 STEC bacteria are not detected are tested for Shiga toxin and cultured for STEC; positive specimens should also be cultured for STEC. In clinical settings, O157 immunoassays are less useful than EIA tests that distinguish between Stx1 and Stx2 for identifying patients at risk for developing severe disease.

Cell Cytotoxicity Assay

The Vero (African green monkey kidney) and HeLa cell lines are very sensitive to Shiga toxin because they have high concentrations of globotriaosylceramides Gb3 and Gb4, the receptors for Shiga toxin in eukaryotic cells. Sterile fecal filtrates prepared from fresh stool specimens or broth enrichments of selected colonies are inoculated onto cells and observed for typical cytopathic effect. Confirmation that the cytopathic effect is caused by Shiga toxin is performed by neutralization using anti-Stx 1 and anti-Stx 2 antibodies. Although very sensitive, this method is not routinely used in most clinical microbiology laboratories because the method requires familiarity with tissue culture technique, the availability of cell monolayers, and specific antibodies. Testing typically takes 48–72 hours [13].

Specialized Diagnostic Methods

Certain specialized diagnostic methods might be used by public health laboratories for patients with HUS and during outbreak investigations. Immunomagnetic separation (IMS) is useful when the number of STEC organisms in a specimen is expected to be small (e.g., in specimens from patients who seek treatment ≥5 days after illness onset, in specimens from asymptomatic carriers, and in specimens that have been stored or transported improperly) [87,88]. IMS beads labeled with O26, O103, O111, O145, or O157 antisera are commercially available. IMS is not approved by FDA for use on human specimens.

Serodiagnostic methods that measure antibody responses to serogroup-specific lipopolysaccharides can provide evidence of STEC infection [89]. No such tests are commercially available in the United States. CDC uses internally validated tests to detect immunoglobulin M (IgM) and immunoglobulin G (IgG) responses to infection with serogroup O157 and IgM response to infection with serogroup O111 in patient sera obtained during outbreak investigations and for special purposes.

Forwarding Specimens and Isolates to Public Health Laboratories

Specimens to Be Forwarded

All O157 STEC isolates growing on selective agar should be subcultured to agar slants and forwarded as soon as possible to the appropriate public health laboratory for additional characterization, in compliance with the recommendations of the receiving laboratory and shipping regulations. If agar slants are not available at the submitting laboratory, an acceptable alternative might be a swab that is heavily inoculated with representative growth and placed in transport medium.

Not all specimens that test positive for Shiga toxin yield an easily identifiable O157 STEC or non-O157 STEC colony on subculture. All Shiga toxin–positive specimens or broths from which no STEC isolate was recovered should be forwarded to the appropriate public health laboratory for isolation and additional testing; shipping of Shiga toxin–positive specimens or broths should not be delayed pending bacterial growth or isolation. Broths that cannot be shipped on the day that the EIA test is performed should be stored at 4°C (3 9°F) until they are prepared for shipping.

Public health laboratories should be prepared to accept isolates and broths for additional testing, with or without the primary stool specimen, that were Shiga toxin–positive in an EIA. Clinical laboratories should contact the appropriate public health laboratory to determine the laboratory's preferences and applicable regulations.

Transport Considerations

United Nations regulations (Division 6.2, Infectious Substances) stipulate that a verotoxigenic *E. coli* culture is a category A (United Nations number 2814) infectious substance, which is an infectious substance in a form capable of causing permanent disability or life-threatening or fatal disease in otherwise healthy humans or animals when exposure to the substance occurs. The International Air Transportation Association (IATA) and Department of Transportation (DOT) have modified their shipping guidance to comply with this requirement [90,91]. Therefore, all possible and confirmed O157 STEC and non-O157 STEC isolates and Shiga toxin– positive EIA broths should be shipped as category A infectious substances. If the identity of the infectious material being transported has not been confirmed or is unknown, but the material might meet the criteria for inclusion in category A (e.g., a broth culture that is positive for Shiga toxin or a stool culture from a patient that might be part of an O157 STEC outbreak), certain IATA regulations apply [91]. Both IATA and DOT require that all persons who package, ship, or transport category A infectious substances have formal, documented training every 2 years [92,93].

Category A substances must be packaged in a water-tight primary receptacle. For shipment, slants or transport swabs heavily inoculated with representative growth are preferred to plates. Plates are acceptable only in rare instances in which patient diagnosis or management would be delayed by subculturing an organism to a slant for transport; shipment of plates must be preapproved by the receiving public health laboratory. If a swab is used, the shaft should be shortened to ensure a firm fit within the plastic sheath, and the joint should be secured with parafilm to prevent leakage. When shipping enrichment broths, the cap must fit tightly enough to prevent leakage into the shipping container, and parafilm should be wrapped around the cap to provide a better seal.

Slants, swabs of pure cultures, and plates (if approved by the receiving laboratory) may be shipped at ambient temperature. Stools in transport media, raw stools, and broths should be shipped with a cold pack to prevent growth of other gram- negative flora.

Commercial couriers vary regarding their acceptance of category A agents; clinical laboratories should check with their preferred commercial courier for current requirements. Shipping category A specimens by commercial couriers usually incurs a surcharge in addition to normal shipping fees. Category A infectious substances are not accepted by the U.S. Postal Service [94].

Shipping by a private (noncommercial) courier that is dedicated only to the transport of clinical specimens does not exempt specimens from DOT or IATA regulations; category A specimens must be packaged according to United Nations Division 6.2 regulations with appropriate documentation, even if not being transported by a commercial carrier [94].

Based on existing specifications, laboratories should collaborate to develop specifications for packaging and shipping, which should be incorporated into a standard operating procedure and followed consistently. A United Nations–approved category A shipping container must be used for cultures, and cultures must be packaged and documented according to DOT and IATA regulations [95].

Interpretation of Final Results

Several tests for clinical or public health microbiology laboratories are available for the detection of STEC, and they may be used alone or in combination. No testing method is 100% sensitive or specific, and the predictive value of a positive test is affected by the patient population that a particular laboratory serves. Specificity and sensitivity might be increased by using a combination of tests. However, when test results conflict, interpretation might be difficult, especially when clinical and public health laboratory test results are compared.

Clinical and public health laboratories document STEC test results in a final report (Table 2). Discordant results (e.g., positive immunoassay at a clinical laboratory but negative PCR result at a public health laboratory) might need to be discussed among the treating physician, public health epidemiologist, and clinical and public health laboratory staff members; however, the outcome of most patients' illnesses (i.e., resolution of symptoms or progression to HUS) is already known by the time the discordant laboratory findings are resolved. Proper interpretation of test results, which is needed for appropriate patient evaluation and treatment, includes consideration of several factors, including whether the type of specimen tested was appropriate for the test (e.g., specimens from rectal swabs or whole stools placed in transport medium), the timing of the specimen collection relative to illness onset, the patient's signs and symptoms, the epidemiologic context of the patient's illness, whether the manufacturer instructions were followed precisely, and the possibility of a false-positive or false-negative test result.

Clinical Considerations

Accurate, rapid identification of STEC, particularly of *E. coli* O157:H7, is critical for patient management and disease control. Therefore, the types of microbiologic tests chosen, performed, and reported and subsequent communication with treating clinicians are critical. Prompt and proper treatment of patients with a positive or presumptively positive STEC culture requires rapid and clear diagnostic enteric microbiology and reporting of data. More detailed information on clinical considerations and care of patients with STEC infection is available from recent clinical reviews [32,96,97].

Conclusion

Accumulated findings from investigations of STEC outbreaks, studies of sporadic STEC infections, and passive and active surveillance provide compelling evidence to support the recommendation that all stools submitted for routine testing to clinical laboratories from patients with community-acquired diarrhea should be cultured for O157 STEC and simultaneously tested for non-O157 STEC with an assay that detects Shiga toxins. These recommendations should improve the accuracy of diagnosing STEC infections, facilitate assessment of risk for severe illness, promote prompt diagnosis and treatment, and improve detection of outbreaks.

Because of the critical impact of time on diagnosis of STEC, treating patients, and recognizing and controlling outbreaks of STEC infections, attempting to isolate O157 STEC and detect other STEC serotypes simultaneously, rather than separately (i.e., conducting a Shiga toxin test to determine whether to culture), is recommended. Performing culture for O157 STEC while simultaneously testing for all STEC serotypes is critical. O157 STEC are responsible for most STEC outbreaks and most cases of severe disease; almost all strains have the virulence genes *stx2* and *eae*, which are associated with severe disease. Detection of O157 STEC within 24 hours after specimen submission to the laboratory helps physicians to rapidly assess the patient's risk for severe disease and to initiate measures to prevent serious complications, such as renal damage and death. Rapid isolation of the infecting organism helps public health officials quickly initiate measures to detect outbreaks and control the spread of infection.

Because of the dynamic nature of the Shiga toxin–converting phages and the potential of decreased diagnostic sensitivity for these pathogens later during infection, future commercial assays that target stable traits might improve diagnostic sensitivity. To facilitate diagnosis and patient management, future methods would also ideally allow for an assessment of the organism's potential to cause severe disease (e.g., related to the presence of *stx2*, certain *stx2* subtypes, and *eae*). Improved isolation methods for non-O157 STEC also are needed. As nucleotide sequences for more STEC strains become available, comparative genomic studies might identify targets that can be used to improve detection, virulence profiling, and isolation strategies.

The Association of Public Health Laboratories, in conjunction with state and federal partners, is developing guidelines for receiving, testing, isolating, and characterizing STEC isolates and specimens in public health laboratories. That document will complement the guidelines in this report and will be available on the APHL website (http://www.aphl.org) by early 2010. Additional information on STEC is available at http:// www.cdc.gov/ecoli.

Acknowledgments

This report is based, in part, on contributions by J. Michael Miller, PhD, CDC; Phillip Tarr, MD, Washington University School of Medicine, St. Louis, Missouri; Frances Tyrell, Georgia Public Health Laboratory, Atlanta, Georgia; the College of American Pathologists, Northfield, Illinois; the U.S. Department of Agriculture Food Safety and Inspection Service, Washington,

DC; the Food and Drug Administration, Silver Spring, Maryland; and the Centers for Medicare & Medicaid Services, Baltimore, Maryland.

References

[1]   CDC. Importance of culture confirmation of Shiga toxin–producing *Escherichia coli* infection as illustrated by outbreaks of gastroenteritis—New York and North Carolina, 2005. *MMWR*, 2006, 55,1042–5.

[2]   Mead, PS; Slutsker, L; Dietz, V. et al. Food-related illness and death in the United States. *Emerg Infect Dis*, 1999, 5, 607–25.

[3]   Johnson, KE; Thorpe, CM; Sears, CL. The emerging clinical importance of non-O157 Shiga toxin–producing Escherichia coli. *Clin Infect Dis*, 2006, 43,1587–95.

[4]   CDC. Laboratory-confirmed non-O157 Shiga toxin–producing Escherichia coli—Connecticut, 2000–2005. *MMWR*, 2007, 56, 29–31.

[5]   Brooks, JT; Sowers, EG; Wells, JG. et al. Non-O157 Shiga toxin–producing *Escherichia coli* infections in the United States, 1983–2002. *J Infect Dis*, 2005, 192, 1422–9.

[6]   O'Brien, AD; Tesh, VL; Donohue-Rolfe, A. et al. Shiga toxin: biochemistry, genetics, mode of action, and role in pathogenesis. *Curr Top Microbiol Immunol*, 1992, 180, 65–94.

[7]   Mead, PS; Griffin, PM. *Escherichia coli* O157:H7. *Lancet*, 1998, 352, 1207–12.

[8]   Rowe, PC; Orrbine, E; Lior, H. et al. Risk of hemolytic uremic syndrome after sporadic *Escherichia coli* O157:H7 infection: results of a Canadian collaborative study. *J Pediatr*, 1998, 132, 777–82.

[9]   Slutsker, L; Ries, AA; Greene, KD; Wells, JG; Hutwagner, L; Griffin, PM. *Escherichia coli* O157:H7 diarrhea in the United States: clinical and epidemiologic features. *Ann Intern Med*, 1997, 126, 505–13.

[10] Griffin, PM; Tauxe, RV. The epidemiology of infections caused by *Escherichia coli* O1 57:H7, other enterohemorrhagic E. coli, and the associated hemolytic uremic syndrome. *Epi Rev*, 13, 60–98,1991.

[11] Manning, SD; Motiwala, AS; Springman, AC. et al. Variation in virulence among clades of *Escherichia coli* O157:H7 associated with disease outbreaks. *Proc Natl Acad Sci*, U S A. 2008,105, 4868–73.

[12] Ethelberg, S; Olsen, KE; Scheutz, F. et al. Virulence factors for hemolytic uremic syndrome, Denmark. *Emerg Infect Dis*, 2004,10, 842–7.

[13] Paton, JC; Paton, AW. Pathogenesis and diagnosis of Shiga toxin–producing *Escherichia coli* infections. *Clin Microbiol Rev*, 1998, 11, 450–79.

[14] Ake, JA; Jelacic, S; Ciol, MA. et al. Relative nephroprotection during *Escherichia coli* O1 57:H7 infections: association with intravenous volume expansion. *Pediatrics*, 2005, 115, e673–80.

[15] Pollock, KG; Stewart, A; Beattie, TJ. et al. From diarrhoea to haemolytic uraemic syndrome—when to seek advice. *J Med Microbiol*, 2009,58(Pt 4), 397–8.

[16] Bennett, WE; Jr., Tarr, PI. Enteric infections and diagnostic testing. *Curr Opin Gastroenterol*, 2009, 25, 1–7.

[17] Klein EJ; Stapp JR; Clausen CR. et al. Shiga toxin–producing *Escherichia coli* in children with diarrhea: a prospective point-of-care study. *J Pediatr*, 2002, 141, 172–7.

[18] Cohen, MB. Shiga toxin–producing *E. coli*: two tests are better than one. *J Pediatr*, 2002,141,155–6.

[19] Boerlin, P; McEwen, SA; Boerlin-Petzold, F; Wilson, JB; Johnson, RP; Gyles, CL. Associations between virulence factors of Shiga toxin–producing *Escherichia coli* and disease in humans. *J Clin Microbiol*, 1999, 37, 497–503.

[20] Jenkins, C; Willshaw, GA; Evans, J. et al. Subtyping of virulence genes in verocytotoxin-producing *Escherichia coli* (VTEC) other than serogroup O157 associated with disease in the United Kingdom. *J Med Microbiol*, 2003, 52(Pt 11), 941–7.

[21] Werber, D; Fruth, A; Buchholz, U. et al. Strong association between Shiga toxin–producing *Escherichia coli* O157 and virulence genes stx2 and eae as possible explanation for predominance of serogroup O157 in patients with haemolytic uraemic syndrome. *Eur J Clin Microbiol Infect Dis*, 2003, 22, 726–30.

[22] Ostroff, SM; Tarr, PI; Neill, MA. et al. Toxin genotypes and plasmid profiles as determinants of systemic sequelae in *Escherichia coli* O157:H7 infections. *J Infect Dis*, 1989, 160, 994–8.

[23] Andreoli, SP; Trachtman, H; Acheson, DW; Siegler, RL; Obrig, TG. Hemolytic uremic syndrome: epidemiology, pathophysiology, and therapy. *Pediatr Nephrol*, 2002, 17, 293–8.

[24] Bégué, RE; Neill, MA; Papa, EF; Dennehy, PH. A prospective study of Shiga-like toxin-associated diarrhea in a pediatric population. *J Pediatr Gastroenterol Nutr*, 1994, 19, 164–9.

[25] Bokete, TN; O'Callahan, CM; Clausen, CR. et al. Shiga-like toxin–producing *Escherichia coli* in Seattle children: a prospective study. *Gastroenterology*, 1993, 105, 1724–31.

[26] Denno DM; Stapp JR; Boster DR. et al. Etiology of diarrhea in pediatric outpatient settings. *Pediatr Infect Dis J*, 2005, 24, 142–8.

[27] Klein, EJ; Boster, DR; Stapp, JR. et al. Diarrhea etiology in a children's hospital emergency department: a prospective cohort study. *Clin Infect Dis*, 2006, 43, 807–13.

[28] Nataro, JP; Mai, V; Johnson, J. et al. Diarrheagenic *Escherichia coli* infection in Baltimore, Maryland, and New Haven, Connecticut. *Clin Infect Dis*, 2006, 43, 402–7.

[29] Park, CH; Gates, KM; Vandel, NM; Hixon DL. Isolation of Shiga-like toxin producing *Escherichia coli* (O157 and non-O157) in a community hospital. *Diagn Microbiol Infect Dis*, 1996, 26, 69–72.

[30] Gavin, PJ; Peterson, LR; Pasquariello, AC. et al. Evaluation of performance and potential clinical impact of ProSpecT Shiga toxin *Escherichia coli* microplate assay for detection of Shiga toxin–producing *E. coli* in stool samples. *J Clin Microbiol*, 2004, 42, 165–6.

[31] Kehl, K; Havens, P; Behnke, CE; Acheson DW. Evaluation of the premier EHEC assay for detection of Shiga toxin–producing Escherichia coli. *J Clin Microbiol*, 1997, 35, 2051–4.

[32] Tarr, PI; Gordon, CA; Chandler, WL. Shiga toxin–producing *Escherichia coli* and haemolytic uraemic syndrome. *Lancet*, 2005, 365,1073–86.

[33] Jelacic, JK; Damrow, T; Chen, GS. et al. Shiga toxin–producing *Escherichia coli* in Montana: bacterial genotypes and clinical profiles. *J Infect Dis*, 2003, 188, 719–29.

[34] Griffin, PM; Ostroff, SM; Tauxe, RV. et al. Illnesses associated with *Escherichia coli* O157:H7 infections. *Ann Intern Med*, 1988, 109, 705–12.

[35] Griffin, PM; Olmstead, LC; Petras RE. *Escherichia coli* O157:H7-associated colitis. *Gastroentrol*, 1990, 99, 142–9.

[36] Swaminathan, B; Barrett, TJ; Hunter, SB; Tauxe, RV. CDC PulseNet Task Force. PulseNet: the molecular subtyping network for foodborne bacterial disease surveillance, United States. *Emerg Infect Dis*, 2001, 7, 382–9.

[37] De Boer, E; Heuvelink, AE. Methods for the detection and isolation of Shiga toxin–producing *Escherichia coli*. *Symp Ser Soc Appl Microbiol*, 2000, 133S–43.

[38] Dundas, S; Todd, WT; Stewart, AI; Murdoch, PS; Chaudhuri, AK; Hutchinson, SJ. The central Scotland *Escherichia coli* O157:H7 outbreak: risk factors for the hemolytic uremic syndrome and death among hospitalized patients. *Clin Infect Dis*, 2001, 33, 923–31.

[39] Guerrant, RL; Van Gilder, T; Steiner, TS. et al. Practice guidelines for the management of infectious diarrhea. *Clin Infect Dis*, 2001, 32, 331–50.

[40] Shah, S; Hoffman, R; Shillam, P; Wilson, B. Prolonged fecal shedding of *Escherichia coli* O157:H7 during an outbreak at a day care center. *Clin Infect Dis*, 1996, 23, 835–6.

[41] Ahn, CK; Klein, E; Tarr, PI. Isolation of patients acutely infected with *Escherichia coli* O157:H7: low-tech, highly effective prevention of hemolytic uremic syndrome. *Clin Infect Dis*, 2008, 46, 1197–9.

[42] Parry, SM; Salmon, RL. Sporadic STEC O157 infection: secondary household transmission in Wales. *Emerg Infect Dis*, 1998, 4, 657–61.

[43] Carter, AO; Borczyk, AA; Carlson, JA. et al. A severe outbreak of *Escherichia coli* O157:H7–associated hemorrhagic colitis in a nursing home. *N Engl J Med*, 1987, 317,1496–500.

[44] Belongia EA; Osterholm MT; Soler JT; Ammend DA; Braun JE; MacDonald, KL. Transmission of *Escherichia coli* O157:H7 infection in Minnesota child day-care facilities. *JAMA*, 1993, 269, 883–8.

[45] Hedberg, CW; Greenblatt, JF; Matyas, BT. et al. Timeliness of enteric disease surveillance in 6 U.S. states. *Emerg Infect Dis*, 2008, 14, 311–3.

[46] Smith, KE; Stenzel, SA; Bender, JB. et al. Outbreaks of enteric infectious caused by multiple pathogens associated with calves at a farm day camp. *Pediatr Infect Dis J*, 2004, 23, 1098–104.

[47] Proctor, ME; Kurzynski, T; Koschmann, C; Archer, JR; Davis, JP. Four strains of *Escherichia coli* O157:H7 isolated from patients during an outbreak of disease associated with ground beef: importance of evaluating multiple colonies from an outbreak-associated product. *J Clin Microbiol*, 2002, 40, 1530–3.

[48] Karch H; Tarr PI; Bielaszewska, M. Enterohaemorrhagic *Escherichia coli* in human medicine. *Int J Med Microbiol*, 2005, 295, 405–18.

[49] van Duynhoven, YT; Friesema, IH; Schuurman, T. et al. Prevalence, characterisation and clinical profiles of Shiga toxin–producing *Escherichia coli* in The Netherlands. *Clin Microbiol Infect*, 2008,14, 437–45.

[50] Manning, SD; Madera, RT; Schneider, W. et al. Surveillance for Shiga toxin–producing *Escherichia coli*, Michigan, 2001–2005. *Emerg Infect Dis*, 2007,13, 318–21.

[51] Paton, AW; Paton, JC. Detection and characterization of Shiga toxigenic *Escherichia coli* by using multiplex PCR assays for stx1, stx2, eaeA, enterohemorrhagic *E. coli* hlyA, rfbO111, and rfbO157. *J Clin Microbiol*, 1998, 36, 598–602.

[52] CDC. FoodNet surveillance report for 2004 (final report). Atlanta, GA: CDC; 2006. Available at http://www.cdc.gov/foodnet/annual/2004/report.pdf.

[53] Bielaszewska, M; Middendorf, B; Köck, R. et al. Shiga toxin-negative attaching and effacing Escherichia coli: distinct clinical associations with bacterial phylogeny and virulence traits and inferred in-host pathogen evolution. *Clin Infect Dis*, 2008, 47, 208–17.

[54] Bielaszewska, M; Dobrindt, U; Gärtner, J. et al. Aspects of genome plasticity in pathogenic *Escherichia coli. Int J Med Microbiol*, 2007, 297, 625–39.

[55] Tarr, PI; Neill, MA; Clausen, CR; Watkins, SL; Christie, DL; Hickman RO. *Escherichia coli* O157:H7 and the hemolytic uremic syndrome: importance of early cultures in establishing the etiology. *J Infect Dis*, 1990,162, 553–6.

[56] Olesen, B; Jensen, C; Olsen, K; Fussing ,V; Gerner-Smidt, P; Scheutz, F. VTEC O117:K1:H7. A new clonal group of *E. coli* associated with persistent diarrhoea in Danish travellers. Scand, *J Infect Dis*, 2005, 37, 288–94.

[57] Bielaszewska, M; Köck, R; Friedrich, AW; von Eiff, C. et al. Shiga toxin- mediated hemolytic uremic syndrome: time to change the diagnostic paradigm? *PLoS ONE*, 2007, 2, e1024.

[58] Cornick, NA; Jelacic, S; Ciol, MA; Tarr, PI. *Escherichia coli* O157:H7 infections: discordance between filterable fecal Shiga toxin and disease outcome. *J Infect Dis*, 2002, 186, 57–63.

[59] CDC. Clinical Laboratory Improvement Amendments. Subpart K: quality systems for nonwaived testing. Sect. 493.1253: Standard: establishment and verification of performance specifications (2004). Available at http://wwwn.cdc.gov/clia/regs/subpart_k.aspx#493.1253.

[60] March, SB; Ratnam, S. Sorbitol-MacConkey medium for detection of *Escherichia coli* O157:H7 associated with hemorrhagic colitis. *J Clin Microbiol*, 1986, 23, 869–72.

[61] Church, DL; Emshey, D; Semeniuk, H; Lloyd, T; Pitout, JD. Evaluation of BBL CHROMagar O157 versus sorbitol-MacConkey medium for routine detection of *Escherichia coli* O157 in a centralized regional clinical microbiology laboratory. *J Clin Microbiol*, 2007, 45, 3098–100.

[62] Zadik, PM; Chapman, PA; Siddons CA. Use of tellurite for the selection of verocytotoxigenic *Escherichia coli* O157. *J Med Microbiol*, 1993, 39, 15 5–8.

[63] March, SB; Ratnam, S. Latex agglutination test for detection of *Escherichia coli* serotype O157. *J Clin Microbiol,* 1989, 27, 1675–7.

[64] Corbel, MJ. Recent advances in the study of Brucella antigens and their serological cross-reactions. *Vet Bull*, 1985, 55, 927–42.

[65] Borczyk AA; Harnett N; Lombos M; Lior H. False-positive identification of *Escherichia coli* O157 by commercial latex agglutination tests. Lancet 1990;336:946–7.

[66] Bettelheim, KA; Evangelidis, H; Pearce, JL; Sowers, E; Strockbine, NA. Isolation of a Citrobacter freundii strain which carries the *Escherichia coli* O157 antigen. *J Clin Microbiol*, 1993, 31, 760–1.

[67] Blom, M; Meyer, A; Gerner-Smidt, P; Gaarslev, K; Espersen, F. Evaluation of Statens Serum Institut enteric medium for detection of enteric pathogens. *J Clin Microbiol*, 1999, 37, 2312–6.

[68] CDC. Laboratory confirmed Shigella isolates reported to the CDC by species, serotype, and year for 1991–2005. Available at http://www.cdc. gov/ncidod/dbmd/phlisdata/shigtab/2005/shigellatable6_2005.pdf.

[69] College of American Pathologists. Accreditation and laboratory improvement. Available at http://www.cap.org/apps/ cap.portal?_nfpb=true&_ pagelabel=accreditation.

[70] American Proficiency Institute. Available at http://api-pt.com.

[71] Fey, PD; Wickert, RS; Rupp, ME; Safranek, TJ; Hinrichs, SH. Prevalence of non-O157:H7 Shiga toxin–producing *Escherichia coli* in diarrheal stool samples from Nebraska. *Emerg Infect Dis*, 2000, 6, 530– 3.

[72] Park, CH; Kim, HJ; Hixon, DL; Bubert, A. Evaluation of the Duopath Verotoxin test for detection of Shiga toxins in cultures of human stools. *J Clin Microbiol*, 2003, 41, 2650–3.

[73] Starr, M; Bennett-Wood, V; Bigham, AK. et al. Hemolytic-uremic syndrome following urinary tract infection with enterohemorrhagic Escherichia coli: case report and review. *Clin Infect Dis*, 1998, 27, 310–5.

[74] Strockbine, NA; Bopp, CA; Barrett, TJ. Overview of detection and subtyping methods. In: *Escherichia coli* O157:H7 and other Shiga toxin–

producing *E. coli* strains. Kaper JB, O'Brien AD, eds. Washington, DC: American Society for Microbiology, 1998.

[75] CDC. University outbreak of calicivirus infection mistakenly attributed to Shiga toxin-producing *Escherichia coli* O157:H7—Virginia, 2000. *MMWR*, 2001,50, 489–91.

[76] Reischl, U; Youssef, MT; Kilwinski, J. et al. Real-time fluorescence PCR assays for detection and characterization of Shiga toxin, intimin, and enterohemolysin genes from Shiga toxin–producing *Escherichia coli*. *J Clin Microbiol*, 2002, 40, 2555–65.

[77] El Sayed Zaki, M; El-Adrosy, H. Diagnosis of Shiga toxin producing *Escherichia coli* infection, contribution of genetic amplification technique. *Microbes Infect*, 2007, 9, 200–3.

[78] Pulz, M; Matussek, A; Monazahian, M. et al. Comparison of a Shiga toxin enzyme-linked immunosorbent assay and two types of PCR for detection of Shiga toxin–producing *Escherichia coli* in human stool specimens. *J Clin Microbiol*, 2003, 41, 4671–5.

[79] Perelle, S; Dilasser, F; Grout, J; Fach, P. Detection by 5'-nuclease PCR of Shiga-toxin producing *Escherichia coli* O26, O55, O91, O103, O111, O113, O145 and O157:H7, associated with the world's most frequent clinical cases. *Mol Cell Probes*, 2004,18,185–92.

[80] Perelle, S; Dilasser, F; Grout, J; Fach, P. Detection of *Escherichia coli* serogroup O103 by real-time polymerase chain reaction. *J Appl Microbiol*, 2005, 98, 1 162–8.

[81] Guion, CE; Ochoa, TJ; Walker, CM; Barletta, F; Cleary, TG. Detection of diarrheagenic *Escherichia coli* by use of melting-curve analysis and real-time multiplex PCR. *J Clin Microbiol*, 2008, 46, 1752–7.

[82] Persson, S; Olsen, KE; Scheutz, F; Krogfelt, KA; Gerner-Smidt, P. A method for fast and simple detection of major diarrhoeagenic *Escherichia coli* in the routine diagnostic laboratory. Clin Microbiol Infect, 2007,13, 516–24.

[83] Sloan, LM. Real-time PCR in clinical microbiology: verification, validation, and contamination control. *Clin Microbiol Newsl*, 2007, 29, 87–95.

[84] CDC. Clinical Laboratory Improvement Amendments. Subpart K: quality systems for nonwaived testing. Sect. 493.1236: Standard: evaluation of proficiency testing performance. Available at http://wwwn.cdc.gov/ clia/regs/subpart_k.aspx#493. 1236.

[85] Mackenzie, A; Orrbine, E; Hyde, L. et al. Performance of the ImmunoCard STAT! *E. coli* O157:H7 test for detection of *Escherichia coli* O157:H7 in stools. *J Clin Microbiol,* 2000, 38, 1866–8.

[86] Stapp, JR; Jelacic, S; Yea, YL. et al. Comparison of *Escherichia coli* O1 57:H7 antigen detection in stool and broth cultures to that in sorbitol-MacConkey agar stool cultures. *J Clin Microbiol,* 2000, 38, 3404–6.

[87] Chapman, PA; Siddons, CA. A comparison of immunomagnetic separation and direct culture for the isolation of verocytotoxin-producing *Escherichia coli* O157 from cases of bloody diarrhoea, non-bloody diarrhoea and asymptomatic contacts. *J Medical Microbiol,* 1996, 44, 267–71.

[88] Karch, H; Janetzki-Mittmann, C; Aleksic, S; Datz, M. Isolation of enterohemorrhagic *Escherichia coli* O157 strains from patients with hemolyticuremic syndrome by using immunomagnetic separation, DNA-based methods, and direct culture. *J Clin Microbiol,* 1996, 34, 516–9.

[89] Tarr PI. *Escherichia coli* O157:H7: clinical, diagnostic, and epidemiological aspects of human infection. *Clin Infect Dis,* 995, 20, 1–8.

[90] Department of Transportation. 49 CFR Parts 171–178. Guide to changes. Transporting infectious substances safely. Federal Register; 2008. Available at https://hazmatonline.phmsa.dot.gov/services/publication_documents/ Transporting%20Infectious%20Substances%20Safely.pdf.

[91] International Air Transport Association. Available at www.iata.org.

[92] Association of Public Health Laboratories. 2008 laboratory learning links. Available at http://www.aphl.org/courses/pages/lll08.aspx.

[93] American Society of Microbiology. Sentinel laboratory guidelines for suspected agents of bioterrorism and emerging infectious diseases. Packaging and shipping infectious substances 2008. Available at http://www.asm.org/asm/files/leftmarginheaderlist/downloadfilename/ 000000001202/ packingandshipping1-08.pdf.

[94] United States Postal Service. Domestic mail manual. Available at http:// pe.usps.com/text/dmm300/dmm300_landing.htm.

[95] International Air Transport Association. DGR packing instructions 650, Annex 4. Available at www.iata.org.

[96] Ahn, CK, Holt, NJ, Tarr PI. Shiga-toxin producing *Escherichia coli* and the hemolytic uremic syndrome: what have we learned in the past 25 years? Adv Exp Med Biol, 2009, 634, 1–17.

[97] American Academy of Pediatrics. Summaries of infectious diseases: *Escherichia coli* diarrhea (including hemolytic uremic syndrome)

[Section 3]. In: Pickering LK, ed. Red Book: 2006 report of the Committee on Infectious Diseases. 27th ed. Elk Grove Village, IL: American Academy of Pediatrics; 2006.

In: Foodborne Illness, E. coli and Salmonella   ISBN: 978-1-62100-052-5
Editors: M. Laskaris and F. Korol   © 2011 Nova Science Publishers, Inc.

Chapter 5

Peanut Outlook: Impacts of the 2008-2009 Foodborne Illness Outbreak Linked to Salmonella in Peanuts

Kelsey Wittenberger and Erik Dohlman

Abstract

Between January and April 2009, a foodborne illness outbreak linked to *Salmonella* resulted in one of the largest food safety recalls ever in the United States. The source of the outbreak was linked to one peanut processor handling less than 2 percent of the U.S. peanut supply, but the scope of the recalls was magnified because the processed peanut products were used as ingredients in more than 3,900 products. Although consumer purchases of peanut-containing products initially slowed as the scope of the recalls spread, retail purchases returned to normal within several months and the total volume of peanuts processed during the 2008/09 (August-July) marketing year increased slightly from that of the previous year. These developments suggest that the recalls will not have a lasting impact on peanut demand and production.

Keywords: Peanuts, *Salmonella*, food safety

Acknowledgments

The authors are grateful to Mark Ash, Linda Calvin, Lewrene Glaser, Fred Kuchler, Janet Perry, Daniel Pick, and Greg Pompelli of the Economic Research Service for their insightful comments and suggestions on this report.We also appreciate the timely effort and helpful review comments made by Tiffany Arthur and Scott Sanford (Farm Service Agency) and Nathan Smith (University of Georgia).We extend gratitude to Linda Hatcher for excellent and precise editing and for support in preparing the manuscript for publication.

Processed Peanut Recalls of 2009 Linked to *Salmonella*

One of the Largest Food Recalls in U.S. History Is Linked to Processed Peanuts

The 2008-09 foodborne illness outbreak linked to processed peanuts caused one of the largest food recalls in U.S. history. From the time the Centers for Disease Control and Prevention (CDC)[1] began tracking these outbreaks in November 2008 to the agency's final report in April 2009, 714 cases of illness were linked to *Salmonella* Typhimurium and may have contributed to 9 deaths (CDC, 2009). The U.S. Food and Drug Administration (FDA) identified two peanut-processing plants owned by the Peanut Corporation of America (PCA) as the source of contamination. Both plants were primarily intermediary processors that sold ingredients to other companies. Most recalled products, such as cakes, candy, cookies, peanut crackers, and ice cream, contained peanut paste or peanut butter. Other products, including pet foods and snack mixes, contained blanched, granulated, or roasted peanuts. Some recalled products were produced in bulk and sold directly to institutions for use or repackaging. Total recalls involved more than 3,900 products from over 200 companies (CDC, 2009; FDA, 2009b).

The cost to consumers and producers from food safety recalls can be large. Direct costs from recalls were primarily borne by manufacturers of processed foods rather than by manufacturers typically associated with the peanut industry (such as shellers and peanut processors). U.S. peanut supplies were basically unaffected because recalled products contained less than 2 percent of the peanut supply. Nevertheless, sales of nearly all products containing peanuts declined temporarily as consumers waited for potentially harmful products to be identified and removed from store shelves. Initial data suggest that consumer purchases of products containing peanuts declined between January and February 2009 and returned to previous levels by April 2009 (Smith, 2009; The Nielsen Company, 2009a; The Nielsen Company, 2009b; The Nielson Company, 2009c; National Peanut Board, 2009).[2]

Foodborne Illnesses Affect a Wide Range of Products and Can Be Difficult to Trace

An estimated 76 million cases of foodborne illness occur each year in the United States, causing approximately 325,000 hospitalizations and 5,000 deaths (CDC, 2005a). Local and State health departments investigate between 400 and 500 foodborne illness outbreaks each year (CDC, 2005a). These investigations often remain unresolved due to the difficulty of identifying and grouping cases of an outbreak within a short period. In some cases, especially at the start of an investigation, officials are only able to narrow the source of contamination to a particular commodity (such as strawberries) or a group of processors or producers (such as spinach produced in California).

When faced with a large multi-State outbreak and only partial information on the source of contamination, the CDC, along with other regulatory agencies, issues consumer warnings. Recent warnings have involved raw alfalfa sprouts (2009), raw jalapeño peppers and raw serrano peppers (2008), tomatoes (2008), and bagged spinach (2006). As an investigation progresses, regulators are often able to identify the source of contamination more precisely and target their control measures accordingly.

Events Surrounding the 2009 Recalls of Processed Peanuts

CDC first noted a new outbreak of *Salmonella* Typhimurium[3] on November 10, 2008, and worked with State and local partners to assess the outbreak. Preliminary analysis by CDC and public health officials in multiple States through January 4, 2009, suggested peanut butter as the likely source of the bacteria causing the infections (CDC, 2009). On January 8, 2009, the Minnesota Department of Health further identified the likely source as King

Nut peanut butter. The next day, FDA[4] initiated inspections at the processing plant that produced King Nut peanut butter, which was owned by the Peanut Corporation of America (PCA). For a timeline of FDA investigations of PCA processing facilities, see appendix 1.

On January 10, an opened 5-pound container of King Nut peanut butter tested positive for the outbreak strain of *Salmonella*. While it was possible that the peanut butter was contaminated after it was opened, PCA initiated a limited, voluntary recall of King Nut peanut butter. This brand was primarily sold in bulk containers to institutions rather than directly to consumers.

CDC issued 24 public reports about the foodborne disease outbreak from January 8, 2009, to March 16, 2009. CDC began reporting by citing specific recalls:[5] on January 12, CDC issued a public announcement that King Nut peanut butter was the likely source of the outbreak; on January 13, CDC reported further recalls of peanut butter; and on January 16, recalls of peanut crackers were mentioned. However, after initial investigation of PCA's processing plant in Blakely, GA, it became apparent that the recalls would be too numerous to communicate individually in CDC reports.

On January 17, CDC recommended that consumers "postpone eating other peanut butter containing products... until information became available about whether that product may be affected" (CDC, 2009). This report emphasized that major retail brands of peanut butter did not appear to be associated with the outbreak. Furthermore, this report referenced for the first time a standalone FDA website that detailed product recalls associated with peanuts. As this webpage was updated and improved, CDC reports shifted from listing recalled products to referencing product categories and providing a link for more specific information.

PCA, which was headquartered in Lynchburg, VA, processed peanuts in nine production facilities throughout the United States. PCA primarily sold bulk shipments to institutions (cafeterias, nursing homes, etc.) for direct use and to food manufacturers for use as an ingredient in processed foods. The first PCA plant to be investigated by FDA was located in Blakely, GA (appendix 1). Subsequently, several other PCA plants were investigated, and a second processing plant in Plainview, TX, also issued a recall. PCA faced extensive liability as a result of numerous lawsuits filed by consumers and their intermediaries and filed for chapter 7 bankruptcy on February 13, 2009.

The 2008-09 foodborne illness outbreak linked to *Salmonella* in peanuts caused one of the largest food recalls in U.S. history. National news media coverage was more sustained than usual due to the size of the recall and numerous updates. According to the final CDC report published on April 29,

2009, 714 cases of illness linked to *Salmonella* Typhimurium were confirmed, with 9 illnesses contributing to death.

Although peanuts processed by PCA accounted for at most 2 percent of the U.S. peanut supply, they led to the recall of over 3,900 products containing peanuts by more than 200 food manufacturing companies (CDC, 2009; FDA, 2009b). Recalled products containing peanut ingredients include brownies, cakes, pies, many types of candy, cereals, cookies, crackers, donuts, dressings and seasonings, prepared fruit and vegetable products, ice creams, peanut butter and products, pet foods, pre-packaged meals, snack bars, snack mixes, and toppings (FDA, 2009b).

Background on the Peanut Industry

Although relatively small from the perspective of the overall farm economy, peanuts are an important crop in parts of the three main production regions: the Southeast (Georgia, Alabama, Florida, Mississippi, and South Carolina), the Southwest (Texas, Oklahoma, and New Mexico), and the Mid-Atlantic (Virginia and North Carolina). In 2007, 6,182 farms produced peanuts (U.S. Department of Agriculture (USDA), National Agricultural Statistics Service (NASS), 2009b). In 2008/09, production hit a record 5.1 billion pounds with a farm-gate value of $1.2 billion (USDA, NASS, 2009a).[6]

Peanut Processing

The peanut-processing industry is complex, with multiple transactions between firms occurring before the commodity reaches its final market. However, in terms of food safety, the peanut industry is easier to manage than many because peanuts are rarely sold fresh. Processors heat shelled and roasted peanuts to a high temperature, destroying much of the bacteria present. To date, regulation for the control of bacteria has focused on this processing step.

After harvest, raw peanuts are dried to prevent spoilage. USDA provides inspection and grading services, designed to segregate peanuts into edible and inedible classes and to determine quality premiums and producer prices. Often, raw peanuts are then stored in cold storage warehouses until they are further processed.

In the United States, the majority of peanuts are shelled (i.e., the shell is removed) and the majority of shelled peanuts are processed and used as ingredients in peanut butter, snack foods (such as nut and trail mixes), candy, and other products (primarily extracts and flavor enhancers) (figure 1) (appendix 2). A sizable amount of shelled peanuts are also exported and processed in other countries or crushed domestically to obtain peanut oil (used for cooking) and meal (used mainly as an animal feed). In addition, a small amount of peanuts are used as planting seed or roasted and sold as "ballpark" nuts and in-shell snacks.

Large food manufacturers that use shelled peanuts typically process them in-house because they prefer the control and cost savings in-house processing brings. However, some stand-alone processors sell processed peanut ingredients to other food manufacturers. Stand-alone peanut processors, such as PCA, tend to supply a large number of buyers with small batches of processed peanuts.

Prior to the 2009 Recalls, the Volume of Peanut Processing Was Steady

USDA's National Agricultural Statistics Service (NASS) publishes monthly data on peanut stocks and processing, which serve as a proxy for peanut use. Total processing volume was steady between 1999/00 and 2002/03 and then increased for several years until 2004/05. From 2004/05 until 2007/08, volume was steady at around 2.1 billion pounds of "farm stock"[7] peanuts annually as increasing peanut butter processing offset declines in every other category (figure 2). Peanut butter production (and use) was aided by the slow rate of increase in the retail price of peanut butter between 1999 and 2008. Retail peanut butter prices lagged behind the overall Consumer Price Index for much of this decade,[8] particularly after passage of the Farm Security Act of 2002, which loosened supply restrictions and lowered farm-level prices (figure 3) (U.S. Bureau of Labor Statistics (BLS), 2009; Dohlman et al., 2004; Dohlman et al., 2006). The average price of retail creamy peanut butter increased 9 percent between 2007/08 and 2008/09, although prices began to decline following the recalls of peanut products.

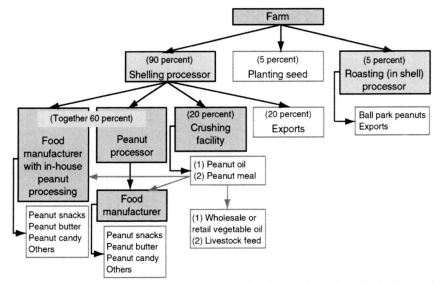

Source: USDA, Economic Research Service, *Oil Crops Outlook*; USDA, National Agricultural Statistics Service, *Peanut Stocks and Processing*; USDA, Foreign Agricultural Service, Global Agricultural Trade System.

Figure 1. An overview of peanut processing.

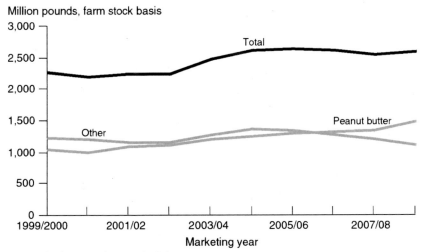

Note: Marketing year is August-July.
Source: USDA, National Agricultural Statistics Service, *Peanut Stocks and Processing.*

Figure 2. Aided by increasing peanut butter processing, total peanut processing increased between 1999/2000 and 2008/2009.

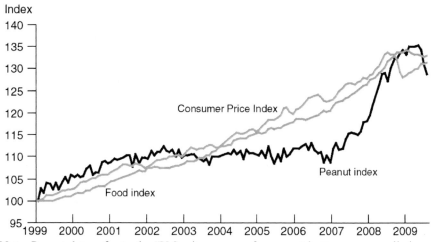

Note: Peanut data refer to the "U.S. city average for peanut butter, creamy, all sizes, per pound." Source: U.S. Department of Labor, Bureau of Labor Statistics.

Figure 3. Retail creamy peanut butter prices trailed overall inflation between 2003 and 2008.

Economic Implications of Peanut Product Recalls

U.S. Federal or State agencies have initiated only two recalls of peanut products, and both recalls were linked to *Salmonella*. The first such recall was due to a foodborne illness outbreak linked to *Salmonella* (serotype Tennessee) in peanut butter in late 2006 through 2007. The source was traced to a single processing facility that produced Peter Pan peanut butter for retail distribution. The peanut processor issued a nationwide, voluntary recall, and FDA, in conjunction with CDC, warned the public. Retailers and consumers were able to identify affected products by the brand name and serial number on the packaging. The identified processing facility was temporarily closed and repaired.

The voluntary recall of peanut butter and consumer warnings in 2007 did not appear to strongly affect use of peanut products. In fact, the primary effect was to increase peanut butter production in order to replace destroyed peanut butter and replenish retail supplies (figure 4). The ease of identification (by brand and batch number) helped consumers and retailers to remove contaminated products and may have contributed to a temporary shift to other brands of peanut butter.

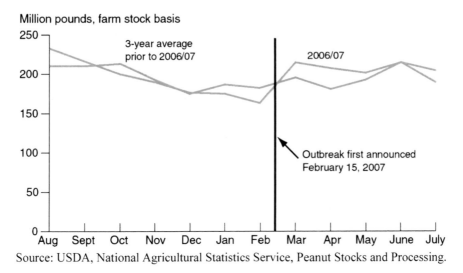

Source: USDA, National Agricultural Statistics Service, Peanut Stocks and Processing.

Figure 4. Peanut processing increased for several months following the 2007 recall of Peter Pan peanut butter.

Economic Implications of 2009 Peanut Product Recalls

Two major companies that collect retail scanner data[9] released 4-week data on peanut butter purchases covering periods during and after the food safety recalls.[10] These data show that 2009 purchases of peanut butter declined in the first 4 weeks of January and February compared with 2008 purchases (Smith, 2009; The Nielsen Company, 2009a; The Nielsen Company, 2009b; The Nielson Company, 2009c; National Peanut Board, 2009). Purchases declined the most in January, with both companies reporting double-digit declines. During the first 4 weeks of April, May, and June 2009, consumer purchases increased from the year before. Consumer purchases were unusually high in April and May.

Several factors may have influenced the reported temporary decline in consumer purchases in 2009 compared with the same period in 2008. First, monthly retail prices for peanut butter (reported by BLS) between January and March were, on average, 10 percent higher in 2009 than during the same timeframe the preceding year (figure 5). Second, by comparing just 2 years of data, it is unclear whether the monthly variations represented normal variability or whether the changes registered in 2009 were a significant departure from longer term trends. Many factors, including seasonal consumption patterns, discounts and promotions, and general economic conditions can affect demand in a given month. Nevertheless, these data indicate that consumers temporarily reduced purchases during the height of the recall of peanut-containing products. Afterwards, purchases increased substantially when information about recalls was more widely disseminated.

Even though the quantity of products involved in the recalls was large, the amount of peanuts contained in these products was not a significant portion of the U.S. peanut supply. Consequently, the recalls did not represent a signif-icant disruption to the available supply of peanuts.

One indicator of anticipated retail demand for peanut products is peanut-processing activity, which reflects orders from food manufacturers and retailers. Even after the recalls were announced, monthly processing volumes remained largely unchanged from, or even higher than, levels of the previous 3 years (figure 6). Despite the temporary decline in retail consumer purchases, the volume of peanuts processed during the entire 2008/09 marketing year (August/July) increased 1.5 percent from the previous year. Processing of peanut butter increased 9 percent from the previous year, from 1.35 billion pounds to 1.47 billion pounds, possibly because major brands of peanut butter were not recalled. However, the quantity of processed snack peanuts declined 14 percent, from 565 million pounds in 2007/08 (on a farm-stock basis) to 489 million in 2008/09.

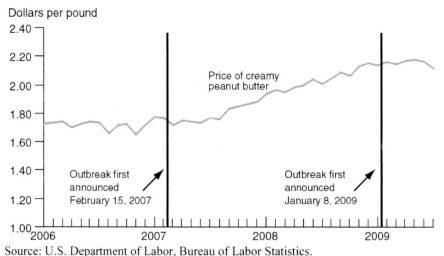

Source: U.S. Department of Labor, Bureau of Labor Statistics.

Figure 5. Recent food safety concerns have not significantly affected peanut butter prices.

While recalls of products containing peanuts did not dramatically affect peanut processing, without the recalls, processing may have increased further for two reasons. First, the 2008 peanut crop was the largest on record. As a result, 2008/09 ending stocks were unusually high and excess supplies might have encouraged greater use. Second, peanut butter is a relatively inexpensive staple good, often cited as "recession proof," and declining consumer incomes might have increased use further in the absence of the recalls.[11] Thus, uncertainty following the recalls of peanut-containing products may have temporarily dampened some of the incentives to further increase peanut processing.

Food safety outbreaks of perishable commodities can have a large effect on the supply and price of available products. In an effort to safeguard the public, regulators can restrict supply and drive up prices. For example, a restriction on imports of green onions in 2004 more than doubled prices for several weeks (Calvin et al., 2004). However, the price of peanut butter following food safety recalls of peanut products in 2009 remained the same as before the recalls (figure 5).[12] Recalls of products containing peanuts were large in total, but did not dramatically restrict supplies of peanut products. In addition, peanut products have a long shelf life, which would help smooth any temporary restriction in supply.[13]

Monthly farm-level peanut prices are another potential indicator of a market reaction to the product recalls (figure 7). Reported farm-level prices actually increased following product recalls; however, the farm-level prices reported by NASS generally do not represent current market conditions. Typically, farmers contract prices before planting begins and may store their harvested peanuts many months before completing a sale to a processor. In addition, a revision to the NASS price-collection methodology (designed to better capture additional payments made to farmers) likely boosted reported prices starting in January 2009.[14]

USDA currently forecasts lower peanut production and prices in 2009/10 than the year before. However, these developments are primarily a response to the large peanut stocks built up by a bumper crop in 2008/09 that was likely far higher than the industry anticipated. With peanut production exceeding anticipated demand by a billion pounds (22 percent of 2008 production),[15] the amount of peanuts in storage at the end of the 2008/09 peanut crop year was near record levels (figure 8).

Responding to the reduced number of peanut contracts and lower contract prices in 2009, farmers planted the lowest number of acres on record since 1915—1.11 million acres. Strong yields should keep production at levels seen in recent years—but production will remain 30 percent lower than in 2008.

Yields for 2009 are favorable because farmers who planted peanuts restricted area to more productive acreage and weather was generally supportive of crop development.

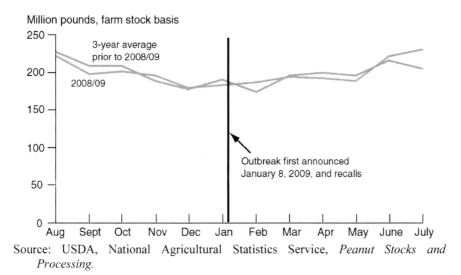

Source: USDA, National Agricultural Statistics Service, *Peanut Stocks and Processing.*

Figure 6. Peanut processing shows little change following 2009 recalls of over 3,900 peanut containing products.

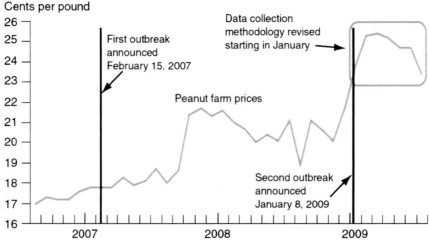

Source: USDA, National Agricultural Statistics Service, Agricultural Prices.

Figure 7. Monthly peanut farm prices appear unaffected by food safety announcements.

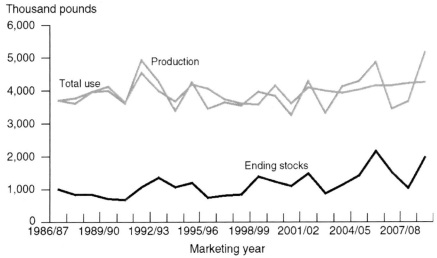

Note: Marketing year is August-July.

Figure 8. Peanut ending stocks rise dramatically in 2008/09.

Current Issues in Food Safety That May Impact the Peanut Industry

In the wake of these and other recent foodborne illness outbreaks, public officials at the national level are considering changes in policies related to prevention, surveillance and enforcement, and response and recovery for all food products.

A number of congressional committee hearings have been held to discuss the outbreak of foodborne illnesses linked to *Salmonella* in peanuts. On February 11, 2009, a congressional hearing by the Oversight and Investigations Subcommittee of the House of Representatives' Committee on Energy and Commerce was held to discuss the outbreak, and industry officials from PCA were issued subpoenas to attend. A subsequent hearing by the same committee on the role of the industry in the outbreak was held on March 19 (Stupak, 2009).

In March, the President created a new Food Safety Working Group, chaired by the secretaries of the U.S. Department of Health and Human Services (HHS) and USDA to review laws and regulations governing food safety (USDA and HHS, 2009). Several steps have been taken to prioritize prevention, strengthen surveillance and enforcement, and improve response and recovery (USDA, 2009).

The national dialogue to re-evaluate food safety laws has been elevated by recent outbreaks linked to *Salmonella* in peanuts and activities of the 111th Congress. On July 30, 2009, the House of Representatives passed the Food Safety Enhancement Act of 2009 (H.R. 2749) (Library of Congress, 2009). A similar version of this bill, the Food Safety Modernization Act (H.R. 875), was referred to the House Agriculture committee and subsequently referred to the subcommittee on Livestock, Dairy, and Poultry (Library of Congress, 2009). The Senate version of the bill (S. 510 - The Food Safety and Modernization Act) was placed on the Legislative Calendar on December 18, 2009.

Conclusions

Costs resulting from 2009 recalls of peanut-containing products were considerable for consumers and producers. The outbreak resulted in at least 714 illnesses, which may have contributed to 9 deaths. In addition, over 3,900 products were recalled by more than 200 companies. U.S. peanut supplies were largely unaffected by these recalls, and the primary concern of the peanut industry was reduced consumer purchases of all products containing peanuts. Retail sales data indicate that, in the months following the initial CDC warning on products containing peanut butter, use declined for several months but returned to previous-year levels 4 months later. The level of peanut processing throughout the outbreak did not diverge significantly from historical trends, suggesting that no major decline in peanut purchases were anticipated going forward.

Nevertheless, the two multistate foodborne illness outbreaks linked to *Salmonella* in peanuts have prompted increased media attention and discussions related to food safety, leading to some new measures enacted by private industry and regulators. During the 2008-09 food recalls linked to peanuts, several trade groups responded by coordinating the flow of information from the peanut industry to consumers and decisionmakers. Individual States, such as Georgia, have also produced legislation to increase oversight of food manufacturing and to establish safety guidelines. At the Federal level, debate in the 111th Congress is focused on the frequency of inspections, on-farm safety standards, preventative safeguards, recall authority, and the organization of public food safety agencies.

The production, supply, and use of peanuts will continue to be governed by fundamental supply and demand prospects. Following a bumper harvest in 2008, ending stocks in 2008/09 were very high. Large ending stocks have already resulted in reduced contracting by peanut shellers in 2009, reducing anticipated prices and lowering the number of planted acres to the lowest level since 1915. Lower production in 2009/10 is forecast to bring ending stocks back to normal, possibly supporting farm-stock peanut prices in 2010. Historically, U.S. per capita peanut consumption has been steady, with overall processing rising at about the rate of population growth (Buzby and Wells, 2009). Peanut-processing increases in 2008/09 (1.5 percent) were similar to historic trend growth despite a temporary slowdown in consumer purchases as a result of the foodborne illness outbreak associated with processed peanuts.

Appendix 1. Investigations by the U.S. Food and Drug Administration of peanut processing plants owned by the Peanut Corporation of America in 2009

Blakely, Georgia	Plainview, Texas
This processing plant primarily produced blanched, split, granulated, and roasted peanuts. Peanut meal, peanut butter, and peanut paste were also produced.	*This processing plant primarily produced peanut butter and peanut paste. Some dry and oil roasted peanuts were also produced.*
January 9—FDA begins preliminary inspections. Production and shipment of peanut paste and peanut butter cease. January 10—PCA voluntarily recalls King Nut and Parnell's Pride peanut butter. January 13—PCA voluntarily recalls certain lots and types of peanut products produced since July 1, 2008. January 16—PCA expands recall to include all peanut butter produced	

Appendix 1. (Continued)

Blakely, Georgia	Plainview, Texas
since August 8, 2008 and all peanut paste produced since September 26, 2008. January 18—PCA expands recall following confirmation of *Salmonella* Typhimurium in unopened peanut butter containers. January 28—FDA completes a preliminary report, which prompts a recall of everything produced since January 1, 2007 (FDA, 2009a). Production at the facility stops. February 5—FDA issues a final investigation report (FDA, 2009a). February 13—PCA files for bankruptcy.	January 21—FDA begins inspections. February 4—Inspectors return to start a comprehensive inspection. February 10—PCA voluntarily ceases production at the request of the Texas Department of State Health Services. February 12—The State of Texas issues an emergency order suspending production and mandating a recall of all products produced since January 1, 2007. February 13—PCA files for bankruptcy. February 26—FDA issues a final investigation report (FDA, 2009a).

Source: Compiled by USDA, Economic Research Service from FDA and CDC websites and personal correspondence.

Appendix 2. Peanuts: Supply and disappearance on a shelled-equivalant basis, United States

| Year beginning Aug. 1 | Supply | | | | Food use | | | | Roasting stock | | Disappearance | | | | | | Price |
	Beginning stocks	Production	Imports	Total	Peanut candy	Snack peanuts	Peanut butter	Other products	Use	Exports	Subtotal	Crush	Exports	Seed use	Shrinkage and residual	Total	Average received by farmers
1986/87	845	3,697	2	4,544	427	511	904	99	139	8	2,073	514	665	219	223	3,694	29.2
1987/88	1,003	3,616	2	4,621	433	497	934	110	112	15	2,072	560	620	226	311	3,789	28.0
1988/89	833	3,981	3	4,817	435	507	1,110	82	132	12	2,255	814	689	227	-12	3,973	27.9
1989/90	843	3,990	4	4,837	439	522	1,193	50	125	7	2,323	624	990	252	-52	4,137	28.0
1990/91	701	3,604	27	4,332	406	472	987	51	111	7	2,021	689	655	277	8	3,650	34.7
1991/92	683	4,927	5	5,615	436	461	1,179	45	101	10	2,211	1,103	1,002	211	33	4,560	28.3
1992/93	1,055	4,284	2	5,341	437	469	1,061	33	135	13	2,122	891	951	216	-189	3,991	30.0
1993/94	1,350	3,392	2	4,744	482	464	967	48	141	14	2,088	670	533	205	188	3,684	30.4
1994/95	1,061	4,247	74	5,382	465	401	944	49	164	14	2,009	982	878	192	123	4,184	28.9
1995/96	1,198	3,461	153	4,812	466	369	968	43	163	16	1,993	999	826	175	61	4,054	29.3
1996/97	758	3,661	127	4,546	480	386	968	44	168	17	2,029	692	668	179	182	3,750	28.1
1997/98	795	3,539	141	4,475	467	408	1,011	47	184	19	2,099	544	682	190	112	3,627	28.3
1998/99	848	3,963	155	4,966	506	465	990	30	181	20	2,153	460	562	192	209	3,576	28.4
1999/00	1,392	3,829	180	5,401	472	524	1,027	27	201	18	2,234	713	743	192	287	4,169	25.4
2000/01	1,233	3,266	216	4,715	473	476	1,002	31	216	15	2,184	548	527	193	167	3,619	27.4
2001/02	1,097	4,277	203	5,577	465	476	1,089	27	180	12	2,226	693	700	169	313	4,101	23.4
2002/03	1,476	3,321	75	4,872	471	459	1,102	32	184	7	2,241	857	490	168	242	3,998	18.2
2003/04	875	4,144	38	5,057	487	551	1,199	22	211	14	2,456	536	516	179	250	3,937	19.3

Year beginning Aug. 1	Supply				Disappearance											Price
	Beginning stocks	Production	Imports	Total	Peanut candy	Snack peanuts	Peanut butter	Other products	Use	Exports	Subtotal	Crush	Exports	Seed use	Shrinkage and residual	Total	Average received by farmers
2004/05	1,121	4,288	37	5,446	518	600	1,248	30	215	12	2,600	393	491	207	340	4,032	18.9
2005/06	1,415	4,870	32	6,317	501	597	1,296	23	216	17	2,616	542	491	155	345	4,150	17.3
2006/07	2,167	3,464	61	5,692	497	552	1,321	13	217	14	2,585	513	603	154	317	4,172	17.7
2007/08	1,520	3,672	73	5,265	426	565	1,346	15	185	21	2,517	496	750	192	279	4,234	20.5
2008/09	1,031	5,162	86	6,279	421	489	1,467	12	212	30	2,571	445	727	139	268	4,149	23.0

Sources: USDA, National Agricultural Statistics Service, U.S. Trade Internet System, and Foreign Agricultural Service, Crop Production, *Peanut Stocks and Processing, and Agricultural Prices.*

References

[1]   Ash, Mark, Erik Dohlman & Kelsey Wittenberger. *Oil Crops Outlook,* Monthly, U.S. Department of Agriculture, Economic Research Service, http://usda.mannlib.cornell.edu/MannUsda/viewDocumentInfo. do?documentID= 1288

[2]   Becker, Geoffrey S. (March 2009). *The Federal Food Safety System: A Primer,* RS22600, Congressional Research Service.

[3]   Buzby, Jean, Laurian Unnevehr & Donna Roberts. (September 2008). *Food Safety and Imports: An Analysis of FDA Import Refusal Reports,* EIB-39, U.S. Department of Agriculture, Economic Research Service, http://www.ers.usda.gov/Publications/EIB39/

[4]   Buzby, Jean & Hodan Farah Wells. (February 2009). Food Availability Data Set, U.S. Department of Agriculture, Economic Research Service, http://www.ers.usda.gov/data/foodconsumption/FoodAvailSpreadsheets. htm#nuts

[5]   Calvin, Linda, Belem Avendano & Rita Schwentesius. (December 2004). *The Economics of Food Safety: The Case of Green Onions and Hepatitis A Outbreaks,* Outlook Report No. VGS-30501, U.S. Department of Agriculture, Economic Research Service, http://www.ers.usda.gov/publications/vgs/nov04/vgs30501/

[6]   Centers for Disease Control and Prevention (CDC). (January 2005a). *Foodborne Illness: Frequently Asked Questions,* http://www.cdc.gov/ncidod/dbmd/diseaseinfo/files/foodborne_illness_F AQ.pdf

[7]   Centers for Disease Control and Prevention (CDC). (May 2008). *Salmonellosis General Information,* http://www.cdc.gov/nczved/dfbmd/disease_listing/salmonellosis_gi.html

[8]   Centers for Disease Control and Prevention (CDC). (February 2009). *Investigation Update: Outbreak of* Salmonella *Typhimurium,* http://www.cdc. gov/salmonella

[9]   Dohlman, Erik, Linwood Hoffman, Edwin Young & William McBride. (June 2006). "The U.S. Peanut Quota Buyout: Sectoral Adjustment to Policy Change Under the 2002 Farm Act," in Blandford, D., and B. Hill, eds., *Policy Reform & Adjustment in the Agricultural Sectors of Developed Countries,* Wallingford, Oxfordshire, UK: CAB International.

[10]   Dohlman, Erik &Janet Livezey. (October 2005). *Peanut Backgrounder,* Outlook Report No. OCS05I01, U.S. Department of Agriculture,

Economic Research Service,
http://www.ers.usda.gov/Publications/OCS/Oct05/OCS05I01/

[11]   Dohlman, Erik, Edwin Young, Linwood Hoffman & William McBride.
       (July 2004). *Peanut Policy Change and Adjustment Under the 2002
       Farm Act,* Outlook Report No. OCS04G01, U.S. Department of
       Agriculture, Economic Research Service,
       http://www.ers.usda.gov/Publications/OCS/Jul04/OCS04G01/

[12]   Frenzen, Paul, Lynn Riggs, Jean Buzby, Thomas Breauer, Tanya
       Roberts, Drew Voetsch & Sudha Reddy. (August 1999). *"Salmonella*
       Cost Estimate Updated Using FoodNet Data," *FoodReview, 22(2),* 10-
       15, http://www.ers.usda.gov/publications/foodreview/may1999/
       frmay99c.pdf

[13]   General Services Administration (GSA) and Office of Management and
       Budget (OMB). (October 2008). *Justification for Non-Substantive
       Change Request - Peanut Prices 2008,*
       http://www.reginfo.gov/public/do/ PRAViewDocument?ref_nbr=2008
       10-0535-00 1

[14]   He, Senhui, W. & Florkowski, A. Elnagheeb. (July 1998). "Consumer
       Characteristics   Influencing   the   Consumption   of   Nut-containing
       Products," *Journal of Food Distribution Research, 28*(2), 31-44.

[15]   He, Senhui, Stanley Fletcher & Arbindra Rimal. (March 2005). "Snack
       Peanut Consumption: Type Preference and Consumption Manners,"
       Journal of Food Distribution Research, 36(1), 79-85.

[16]   Library of Congress. (2009). *Thomas - Home.* The Library of Congress,
       http://thomas.loc.gov/

[17]   National Peanut Board. (September 10, 2009). *We're Going Back to
       Peanut Butter (If We Ever Left It),* http://www.energyforthegoodlife.org/

[18]   The Nielsen Company. February. 2009a. Salmonella *Outbreak Taints
       Peanut   Butter   Sales,*   http://blog.nielsen.com/nielsenwire/tag/peanut-
       butter/

[19]   The Nielsen Company. (March 2009b). *Peanut Butter Sales Still Stuck,*
       http://blog.nielsen.com/nielsenwire/tag/peanut-butter/

[20]   The Nielsen Company. (May 2009c). *Update: Peanut Butter Sales Back
       on Track,* http://blog.nielsen.com/nielsenwire/tag/peanut-butter/

[21]   Smith, Ron. (April 2009). *Peanut Butter Sales Rebound Following*
       Salmonella *Scare,* Southwest Farm Press,
       http://southwestfarmpress.com/peanuts/ peanut-butter-sales-0413/

[22]   Stupak, Bart & Chairman. (March 19, 2009). *The* Salmonella *Outbreak:
       The   Role   of   Industry   in   Protecting   the   Nation's   Food   Supply,*

Congressional hearing, Committee on Energy and Commerce, Oversight and Investigations.

[23] U.S. Bureau of Labor Statistics (BLS). (January 2009). *Consumer Price Index - Average Price Data*, http://www.bls.gov/data/

[24] U.S. Department of Agriculture (USDA). (July 2009). *Obama Administration Delivers on Commitment to Upgrade U.S. Food Safety System*, Press release no. 0292.09.

[25] U.S. Department of Agriculture (USDA) and U.S. Department of Health and Human Services (HHS). (March 2009). *President's Food Safety Working Group*, http://www.foodsafetyworkinggroup.gov/Home.htm

[26] U.S. Department of Agriculture (USDA), Foreign Agricultural Service. Global Agricultural Trade System.

[27] U.S. Department of Agriculture (USDA), National Agricultural Statistics Service (NASS). (February 2009a). *Crop Values 2008 Summary*.

[28] U.S. Department of Agriculture (USDA), National Agricultural Statistics Service (NASS). (February 2009b). (Updated Sept. 2009) *2007 Census of Agriculture*.

[29] U.S. Food and Drug Administration (FDA). (2009a). *Inspectional Observations for the Peanut Corporation of America*, http://www.fda.gov/ora/frequent/ default.htm

[30] U.S. Food and Drug Administration (FDA). (May 2009b). *Peanut Product Recalls:* Salmonella *Typhimurium*, http://www.fda.gov/oc/opacom/hottopics/salmonellatyph.html

End Notes

[1] The food safety role of CDC is primarily to monitor, investigate, and identify foodborne illness outbreaks. It is not a regulatory agency, but it works closely with regulators and health departments at the Federal, State, and local levels to gather information and coordinate communication about risks to the public.

[2] The authors did not have direct access to this retail scanner data. With access to more detailed data, a more refined analysis of consumer purchasing behavior by product type would be possible.

[3] The bacteria *Salmonella* causes the disease salmonellosis in humans, and is the second most common identified foodborne illness for humans in the United States, causing approximately 40,000 cases of salmonellosis each year (CDC, 2008). Because many milder cases are not diagnosed or reported, the actual number of infections is likely much higher, with studies suggesting that less than 1 in 30 Salmonella cases are reported and identified by health professionals (Frenzen et al., 1999).

[4] FDA regulates about 80 percent of the U.S. food supply, with approximately 2,700 food inspection staff throughout the United States responsible for the oversight of roughly 44,000 U.S. food manufacturers and 100,000 registered food facilities (Becker, 2009). Some of the

foods in FDA's purview include dairy products, produce, processed foods, food additives, animal feed, game and exotic meats, and veterinary drugs (Buzby et al., 2008). FDA does not regulate domestic and imported meats, poultry, and processed egg products that are otherwise inspected by USDA's Food Safety and Inspection Service.

[5] All food safety recalls were voluntary and issued by affected companies. FDA coordinated the release of this information, and CDC issued summary reports to more widely communicate this information to the public.

[6] The *Peanut Backg rounder* provides an overview of the policy environment and broad market trends in the peanut industry (Dohlman and Livezey, 2005). The monthly *Oil Crops Outlook* provides up-to-date forecasts of peanut production, supply, demand, and prices (Ash et al., monthly).

[7] USDA adjusts data relating to peanuts to an in-shell-equivalent basis to enable comparison across product categories. A conversion factor of 1.33 is typically used when converting shelled peanuts to an equivalent in-shell measure.

[8] BLS tracks the price of creamy peanut butter in major cities as a part of the Consumer Price Index.

[9] The Nielsen Company and Information Resources, Inc.

[10] Retail sales data are not publicly available for categories of products other than peanut butter. In 2008/09, peanut butter was 57 percent of U.S. peanut processing.

[11] Although the evidence is limited, several studies suggest that peanuts (specifically, snack peanuts) may be, in economics terminology, an "inferior" good. Inferior goods are those for which consumption tends to increase as incomes decline and to decrease as incomes grow (He et al., 2005; He et al., 1998).

[12] BLS does not report sale prices or discounts (coupons) that may have been used to bolster purchases of peanut butter.

[13] A more complete analysis of specific products could help determine the price impacts at a more microeconomic level.

[14] Buyers are now specifically asked the per pound options price they received for contract sales. The options price is a premium paid in addition to the sale price and can be substantial. The change was prompted by concerns by USDA's Farm Service Agency, which reported that NASS prices were incomplete (GSA and OMB, 2008).

[15] USDA 2008/09 total peanut demand forecast as of October 2009.

Chapter Sources

Chapter 1 - This is an edited, reformatted and augmented version of a Congressional Research Service publication, R40916, dated April 15, 2010.

Chapter 2 - This is an edited, reformatted and augmented version of a Congressional Research Service publication, RL33722, dated November 13, 2006.

Chapter 3 - This is an edited, reformatted and augmented version of a US Centers for Disease Control and Prevention FAQ publication, dated June, 2011.

Chapter 4 - This is an edited, reformatted and augmented version of a US Department of Health and Human Services publication, No.RR-12, dated October 16, 2009.

Chapter 5 - This is an edited, reformatted and augmented version of a USDA Economic Research Service Report, OCS-10a-01, dated February, 2010.

Index

G

H

I

T